AF589425

Dedicated to

my late parents
Thiru. N. Pattusamy and Thirumathi. K. Poongavanam
&
My brother **Thiru. N. P. Vertri Kulasekaran**
who has been my inspiration and the
driving force for all my accomplishments
in both Personal and Professional life.

AN OCCUPATIONAL THERAPIST HELPS YOU TO GLITTER WITH THE SHADES THAT YOU OWN

IN THE WORLD OF AN OCCUPATIONAL THERAPIST, CHALLENGES BECOME OPPORTUNITIES

CONTENTS

FOREWORD

It is with great pleasure and enthusiasm that I write this foreword for "Raghuram's Handbook of Occupational Therapy". In the pages that follow, you will embark on a profound exploration of a field that has the power to transform lives, install hope, and empower individuals at every stage of their existence.

As we journey through life, we often encounter moments of vulnerability, challenge, and growth. From the tender moments of infancy, where the world is a place of wonder and discovery, to the twilight years of reflection and wisdom, where each day carries the weight of cherished memories, Occupational Therapy stands as a beacon of support and encouragement.

This comprehensive guide, authored by dedicated professionals with deep-rooted expertise in the field, delves into the heart of Occupational Therapy. It encompasses the full spectrum of human development, recognizing that occupation is not merely a task or an activity but the very essence of our being. Through these pages, you will discover the profound impact that purposeful engagement in occupation can have on one's physical, emotional, cognitive, and social well-being.

"Raghuram's Handbook of Occupational Therapy" is more than a book; it is a testament to the tireless dedication of Occupational Therapists who tirelessly work to enhance the quality of life for individuals, families, and communities. It showcases the profession's commitment to evidence-based practice, holistic care, and the unwavering belief that every individual, regardless of age or circumstance, has the capacity to lead a life of meaning and fulfilment.

Throughout this book, you will find the role and importance of Occupational Therapy. It is a valuable resource for students, practitioners, educators, and anyone seeking to understand about Occupational Therapy.

May this book serve as a guide, and a reminder about Occupational Therapy of the remarkable capacity of the human spirit to adapt, heal, and thrive through the life.

In closing, I extend my deepest appreciation to the authors for their dedication to the field and for sharing their expertise with a wider audience. I commend their commitment to empowering lives, from the very first breath to the twilight years, and I invite you to join them on this extraordinary journey.

May this book inspire you to be an advocate for change, and a beacon of hope for those you serve.

With warm regards,

Dr. Jyothika Nand Bijlani,

Dean, ACOT, AIOTA.

Former Prof & HOD, Occupational Therapy School & Centre,

LTMM College & General Hospital, Mumbai.

PREFACE

In the intricate tapestry of human existence, there lies an art—an art woven into the fabric of daily life, an art that touches every age, every stage, and every soul. It is the art of *Occupational Therapy.*

Welcome to a journey that transcends the boundaries of age, a voyage that explores the boundless potential of occupation, and a celebration of the extraordinary resilience of the human spirit.

Occupational Therapy is more than a career; it's a calling. It's a discipline that enables individuals to regain their independence, adapt to life's challenges, and discover their true potential. This book talks about the role of Occupational Therapy in various fields and its importance.

As you embark on this journey through the pages of our book, we invite you to embrace the vision it holds—an image of a world where occupation is the vehicle for empowerment, where every individual, from the very first breath to the wisdom-filled years, can lead a life of purpose and fulfilment.

We hope that this book serves as a valuable resource for you on your path to becoming an Occupational Therapist or refining your existing skills. May it inspire you to make a positive impact on the lives of those you serve and continue to fuel your enthusiasm for this remarkable profession

May you find inspiration, wisdom, and the courage to make a difference in the lives of those you serve. May you become an artist of occupation, shaping the narratives of countless souls, nurturing their potential, and empowering them to write the most beautiful chapters of their lives.

With heartfelt gratitude for your companionship on this extraordinary journey,

Prof. Raghuram P

ACKNOWLEDGMENT

Writing this Occupational Therapy book has been a labor of love and dedication, and I owe my gratitude to numerous individuals and institutions who have supported me throughout this endeavor.

I extend my appreciation to **Sri Ramachandra Institute of Higher Education and Research (DU)** for their resources, facilities, and the opportunity that has contributed to the content of this book. I am grateful to our respected **Chancellor, Pro- Chancellor, Vice - Chancellor, Pro - Vice Chancellor** for their support.

I value our **Ex- Vice - Chancellor Dr. P.V. Vijayaraghavan** for his valuable support. And also the current **Additional Register Dr. S. Senthil Kumar** for his mentorship and continous guidance and support. I thank the **Chief Librarian, SRIHER Dr. P. Sankar** for his valuable support. Extending my thanks to **Mr. L. Bhaskaran, Superintendent, Administration, SRIHER** for his continous support. I thank the Office Bearers of All India Occupational Therapists' Association (AIOTA).

I am profoundly thankful to my mentors and colleagues in the field of Occupational Therapy who have provided guidance, shared their expertise, and challenged me to strive for excellence. Your wisdom has been invaluable.

To the patients and their families who have entrusted me with their care, I am deeply grateful. Your resilience, courage, and stories have inspired my commitment to advancing Occupational Therapy knowledge.

My dedicated research team deserves special recognition for their tireless efforts in collecting and analyzing data, as well as for their contributions to the research that underpins this book.

My family and friends have provided unwavering support, understanding, and encouragement during long hours of research and writing.

I want to acknowledge the pioneering researchers and Occupational Therapy professionals whose work has inspired me throughout my career. Your dedication to improving healthcare has been a guiding light.

I want to thank **SRIHER – SRFOT Batch 2017 (Phoenix'17), Dr. Shalini (Batch 2017) and Zorticanz (Batch 2018)** for their valuable input.

This book is a testament to the collective efforts and collaboration of these remarkable individuals and institutions. I am truly humbled by your support and grateful for the opportunity to contribute to the field of medicine.

- Prof. Raghuram P

AUTHORS AND CONTRIBUTORS

Author:

Prof. Raghuram P,
Head, Sri Ramachandra Faculty of Occupational Therapy (SRFOT),
Sri Ramachandra Institute of Higher Education and Research (SRIHER),
Porur, Chennai.

Co-Authors:

Dr. Jose Mary Sangeetha. X (OT)
Occupational Therapist,
Department of Physical Medicine Rehabilitation (PMR)
JIPMER (Govt. Of. India),
Puducherry.

Dr. Loganathan S (OT),
Assistant Professor,
Sri Ramachandra Faculty of Occupational Therapy (SRFOT),
Sri Ramachandra Institute of Higher Education and Research (SRIHER),
Porur, Chennai.

Dr. T Sundaresan (OT),
Assistant Professor,
Sri Ramachandra Faculty of Occupational Therapy (SRFOT),
Sri Ramachandra Institute of Higher Education and Research (SRIHER),
Porur, Chennai.

Contributors:

Dr. Vinoth Kumar T (OT),
Faculty, Sri Ramachandra Faculty of Occupational Therapy (SRFOT),
Sri Ramachandra Institute of Higher Education and Research (SRIHER),
Porur, Chennai.

Ms. Kiruthika K,
(Master of Occupational Therapy - Neurology),
Sri Ramachandra Faculty of Occupational Therapy (SRFOT),
Sri Ramachandra Institute of Higher Education and Research (SRIHER),
Porur, Chennai.

Ms. Monisha T,
(Master of Occupational Therapy - Paediatrics),
Sri Ramachandra Faculty of Occupational Therapy (SRFOT),
Sri Ramachandra Institute of Higher Education and Research (SRIHER),
Porur, Chennai.

Ms. Sweatha I,
(Master of Occupational Therapy - Paediatrics),
Sri Ramachandra Faculty of Occupational Therapy (SRFOT),
Sri Ramachandra Institute of Higher Education and Research (SRIHER),
Porur, Chennai.

Ms. Uvanthiga E,
(Master of Occupational Therapy - Paediatrics),
Sri Ramachandra Faculty of Occupational Therapy (SRFOT),
Sri Ramachandra Institute of Higher Education and Research (SRIHER),
Porur, Chennai.

Mr. Lokesh Kumar M N
(Master of Occupational Therapy - Hand and Musculoskeletal Rehabilitation),
Sri Ramachandra Faculty of Occupational Therapy (SRFOT),
Sri Ramachandra Institute of Higher Education and Research (SRIHER),
Porur, Chennai.

Chapter 1

INTRODUCTION

What is Occupational Therapy?

Occupational Therapy is a healthcare profession that focuses on helping individual's to participate in meaningful and purposeful daily activities, known as "Occupations." These occupations encompass a wide range of activities, including self-care tasks (e.g., dressing, grooming, eating), work-related activities, leisure and recreational pursuits, and activities that are essential for community participation.

Who is an Occupational Therapist?

Occupational Therapists are licensed and highly trained professionals who work with people facing physical, cognitive, emotional, or developmental challenges that may affect their ability to engage in these daily activities. The primary goal of Occupational Therapy is to enable individuals to lead fulfilling and independent lives by improving their functional abilities, enhancing their quality of life, and promoting overall well-being.

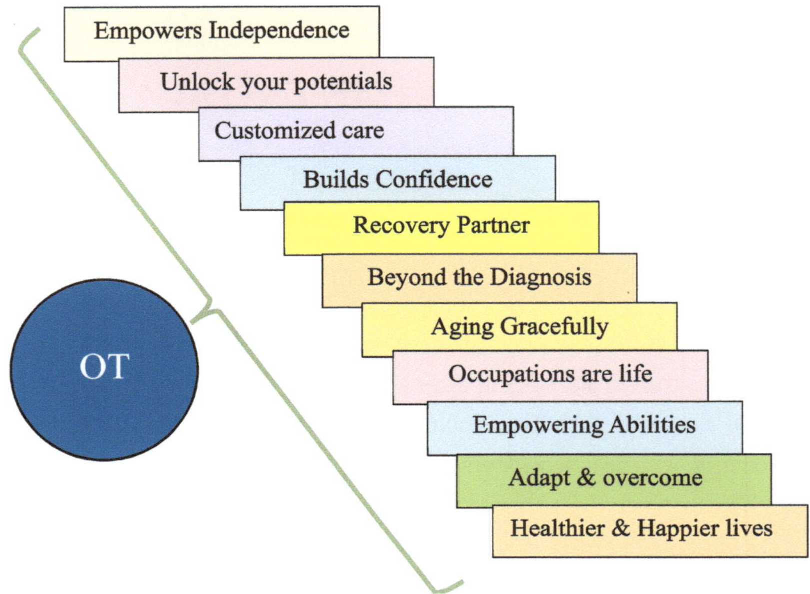

Key aspects of Occupational Therapy include:

- **Holistic Approach:** Occupational Therapists view the whole person, considering their physical, cognitive, emotional, social, and environmental factors. This holistic perspective helps to identify barriers for participation and guides intervention plans.
- **Individualized Care:** Occupational Therapy is highly individualized, with therapists tailoring their approaches to the unique needs, goals, and preferences of each client.
- **Assessment:** Occupational Therapists conduct comprehensive assessments to evaluate a person's strengths, limitations, and areas of concern. These assessments help to identify specific challenges and areas where improvement is needed.

- **Intervention:** Occupational Therapists use a wide range of therapeutic techniques and strategies to address challenges and improve functional abilities. This can include activities, adaptive equipment recommendations, cognitive rehabilitation, sensory integration, and more.
- **Prevention:** Occupational Therapists work on preventive measures, such as fall prevention strategies for older adults, ergonomic assessments to reduce workplace injuries, health and wellness programs related to prevention.
- **Advocacy:** Occupational Therapist advocate for their clients needs, collaborating with healthcare teams, families, educators, and other professionals to ensure individuals receive the support and accommodations they require.
- **Age Group and Population:** Occupational Therapy serves people of all ages, from infants and children with developmental delays to adults recovering from injuries or living with chronic conditions to seniors striving to manage functional independence.
- **Settings:** Occupational Therapists work in various settings, including hospitals, rehabilitation centres, schools, mental health facilities, nursing homes, community health centers, and private practices.
- **Conditions Addressed:** Occupational Therapist help individuals with a wide range of conditions, including physical injuries, neurological disorders, mental health conditions, developmental disorder, and more.
- **Promotion of Participation:** The goal of Occupational Therapy is to promote active participation in daily life activities, empowering individuals to overcome challenges, adapt to their environments, and lead fulfilling lives.

Summary

Occupational Therapy is a client-centred profession that empowers individuals to achieve their goals, regain or enhance their functional independence, and live life to the fullest. By focusing on meaningful occupations, Occupational Therapy help people not only improve their physical and mental health but also fosters a sense of purpose and fulfilment in their Quality of life.

HEALTH CARE TEAM MEMBERS

- ☐ Physiatrist
- ☐ Orthopedic surgeon
- ☐ Neurologist
- ☐ Neurosurgeon
- ☐ Plastic surgeon
- ☐ Psychiatrist
- ☐ Pediatrician
- ☐ Obstetrician
- ☐ Geneticist
- ☐ Neonatologist

- ☐ Rheumatologist
- ☐ Cardiologist
- ☐ Cardiac surgeon
- ☐ General surgeon
- ☐ Oncologist
- ☐ Dermatologist
- ☐ Nephrologist
- ☐ Urologist
- ☐ Ophthalmologist
- ☐ Otorhinolaryngologist
- ☐ Nurse
- ☐ Pharmacologist

- ☐ Occupational Therapist
- ☐ Physiotherapist
- ☐ Speech language pathologist
- ☐ Clinical Psychologist
- ☐ Clinical Nutritionist
- ☐ Medical Social Workers

Chapter 2

HISTORY OF OCCUPATIONAL THERAPY

The history of Occupational Therapy is a fascinating journey that has evolved over time and around the world, and its development has been shaped by various social, cultural, and medical factors.

Here is an overview of the history of Occupational Therapy worldwide.

18th and 19th Centuries

Precursors to Occupational Therapy can be traced back to the 18th century when Quakers and moral treatment advocates in Europe and the United States emphasized the therapeutic value of engaging individuals with mental illness in purposeful activities.

The late 19th-century arts and crafts movement encouraged meaningful and creative activity as a form of healing.

Early 20th Century

The formal roots of Occupational Therapy can be traced to the early 20th century when it was recognized as a profession. The term "Occupational Therapy" was coined by George Edward Barton in 1915.

World War I and World War II played a significant role in the growth of Occupational Therapy. Occupational Therapists were needed to help wounded soldiers regain their independence through purposeful activities.

Eleanor Clarke Slagle is considered one of the founders of Occupational Therapy, and she established the first Occupational Therapy educational program at the University of Southern California in 1942.

Mid-20th Century

In order to serve better for a variety of populations, Occupational Therapy have broadened its focus and started working with kids, people with physical disabilities, and people suffering from mental illnesses. With improvements in medical and psychological care, the profession has evolued widely.

Late 20th Century and Beyond

Occupational Therapy continued to diversify and expand into various settings, including schools, hospitals, rehabilitation centres and private practices.

The World Federation of Occupational Therapists (WFOT) was founded in 1952, promoting global collaboration and standardization within the profession.

Contemporary Occupational Therapy

In recent decades, Occupational Therapy has continued to adapt and innovate, incorporating evidence-based practices and research to improve client outcomes.

Occupational Therapists work with a diverse population, including children with developmental disorders, individuals with mental health disorders, the elderly, and those recovering from injuries or surgeries.

The profession has gained recognition for its role in promoting health and wellness and preventing disabilities through activities and environmental modifications.

Occupational Therapy practitioners play a key role in areas like Rehabilitaion, Assistive Technology, Ergonomics and Community Based Rehabilitation (CBR).

Here is an overview of the history of Occupational Therapy in different parts of the world:

United States:

The roots of Occupational Therapy in the United States can be traced back to the late 19th century. Dr. William Rush Dunton, a psychiatrist, and George Edward Barton, an architect, played pivotal roles in the development of the profession.

Eleanor Clarke Slagle, often referred to as the "Mother of Occupational Therapy," established the first Occupational Therapy training program at the Henry B. Favill School of Occupations in 1915.

OT gained prominence during and after World War I when it was used to rehabilitate injured soldiers. This led to the establishment of the Reconstruction Aides program, which trained women to become OTs.

Canada

Occupational Therapy in Canada has a similar history to that of the United States, with early influences coming from American practitioners. In 1922, the first OT educational program was established at the University of Toronto, setting the stage for the development of OT in Canada.

United Kingdom

Occupational Therapy in the UK has its roots in the moral treatment movement of the 18th and 19th centuries, with a focus on providing meaningful activities to individuals with mental illnesses.

The profession expanded during and after World War I, and the Society of Trained Occupational Therapists (STOT) was established in 1936, which later became the College of Occupational Therapists.

Europe

Occupational Therapy developed independently in various European countries. It was influenced by the work of early proponents in the United States and the UK. European countries gradually established their own professional organizations and educational programs.

Australia and New Zealand

Occupational Therapy in Australia and New Zealand has its origins in the early 20th century. The first Occupational Therapy training programs were established in Australia in the 1930s.

Occupational Therapy in these countries has grown significantly and continues to adapt to the changing healthcare landscape.

India

The founding of the profession of Occupational Therapy in India & Asia came about from the very deep & personal feelings of Mrs. Kamla V. Nimbkar towards her adopted country, India. Mrs. Nimbkar came across an article on Occupational Therapy by Miss Helen Willard, the Head of the Philadelphia School of Occupational Therapy [later joined with the University of Pennsylvania]. Mrs. Nimbkar realized that this was something India did not have but it is much needed.

Thus in 1950 the First school in India & Asia was started at K.E.M. hospital, which received recognition of the World Federation of Occupational Therapy, & became one of their founder members in the year 1952.

During last 50 years Indian Occupational Therapists have nurtured the domain of rehabilitation by productive & pragmatic research. These contributions ensure that the entire profession, its practice kept growing, serving humankind & communicated the essence of its service to the persons with disability to improve their quality of life.

Summary

Throughout its history, Occupational Therapy has evolved from a primarily mental health and rehabilitation-focused field to a diverse profession that addresses the needs of people across the lifespan, from various cultural backgrounds, and in a wide range of settings. Occupational Therapists now work with individuals with physical disabilities, mental health conditions, children with developmental disorders, and the elderly to promote health and well-being through meaningful activities. The profession continues to advance and adapt to meet the evolving needs of society.

Chapter 3

ALL AGES & ALL STAGES

Introduction

"All Ages and All Stages" is a phrase often used to emphasize inclusivity and accessibility, typically in the context of services, activities, or programs that are designed to be suitable for people of all age groups and at all points or stages of life. It signifies that whatever is being offered is intended to be welcoming and relevant to everyone, regardless of their age or life stage.

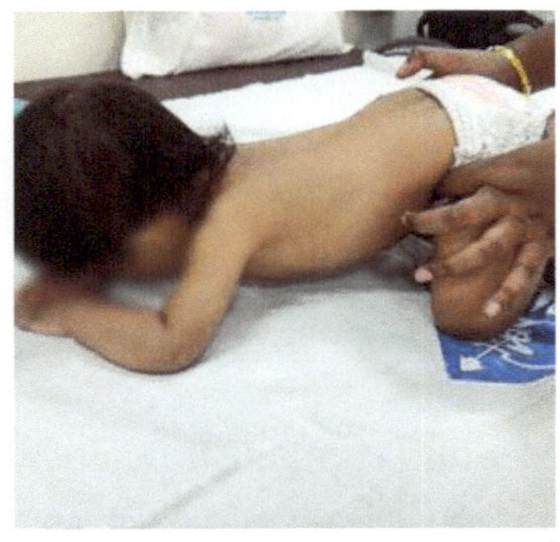

(a) Positioning

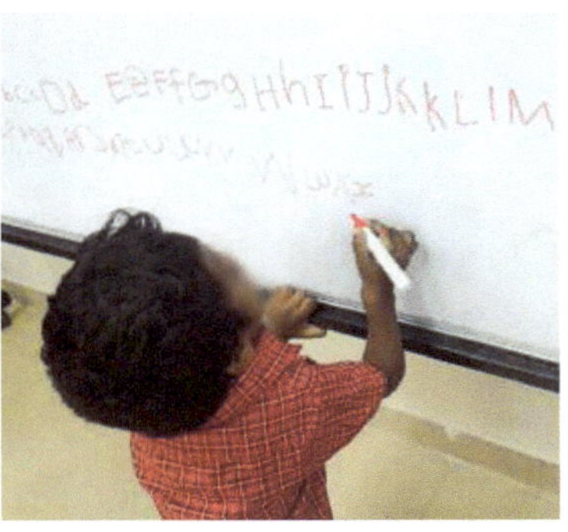

(b) Handwriting training

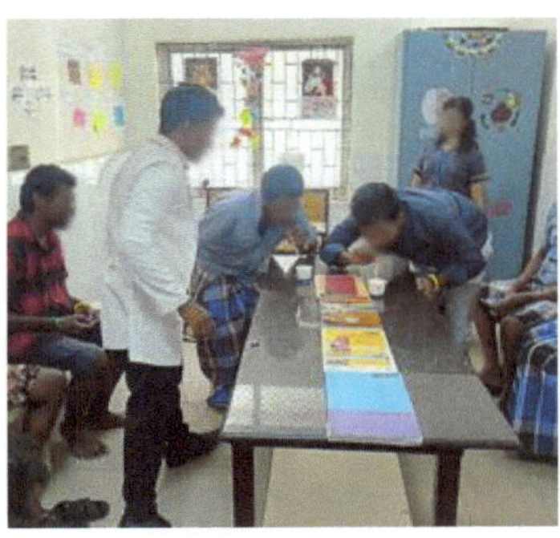

(c) Recreational Therapy

Role of Occupational Therapy in All Ages and All Stages

Occupational Therapy is a healthcare profession focusing on assisting people of all ages and all stages of life to engage in meaningful and useful tasks, or "occupations." Occupational Therapists work with people of all ages in a variety of settings, such as clinics, hospitals, schools, and rehabilitation facilities.

Our role is to be service providers:

- Post-secondary Education/Training
- Independent Living
- Competitive Employment
- Role Competence
- Community Participation
- Well-Being
- Occupational justice

Occupational Therapy for Children

- Occupational Therapist work with infants and young children to address Development Delays, Sensory Processing disorders and Motor Skill development.
- Occupational Therapist help children with Learning Difficulties, improve their fine motor skills, handwriting, academic skills, and social interaction skills.
- Additionally, this service offers programs for assessment, Client centered intervention, and Group Therapy.

Occupational Therapy for Adults

- Assess for and advise on safety measures in the home
- Fall Prevention.
- Building a "dementia-friendly" home.
- Home modification

Occupational Therapy for Geriatrics

- **Dementia Care:** Occupational Therapist specializes in working with dementia patients. Helping them to maintain cognitive function, manage daily routines, and ensure a safe home environment.
- **Home Modifications:** Occupational Therapist assesses and recommends home modifications to enhance safety and accessibility for older adults who wish to age in place.
- **Assistive and Adapive devices:** They provide guidance on selecting and using assistive devices like wheelchairs, walkers, and adaptive utensils.
- **Long-Term Care:** Occupational Therapists provide a variety of therapeutic interventions to raise patients' Quality of Life in homes and assisted living facilities.

Self-Care Activities

Meal Preparation

Home Management

Play & Leisure

Care of others

Financial Management

Social Participation

Community Mobility

Safety Procedures

Summary

Occupational Therapy is a flexible field that helps people of all ages and stages to overcome challenges and engaging in meaningful activities and enhance their general Quality of Life. Occupational Therapist employs a client-centred methods to customize interventions to the needs and objectives of each person with whom they work.

CHAPTER 4

OBSTETRICS AND GYNAECOLOGY

Introduction

Occupational Therapists play a valuable role in the field of Obstetrics and Gynecology (OBGYN) by addressing the unique physical and psychological needs of individuals during pregnancy, labor, and the postpartum period.

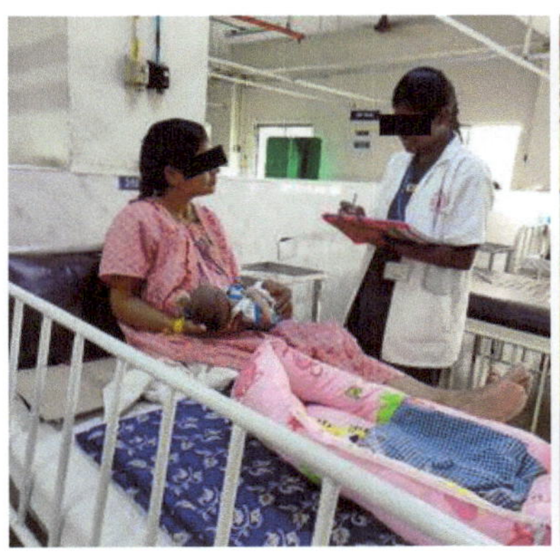

(a) **Postpartum Assessment**

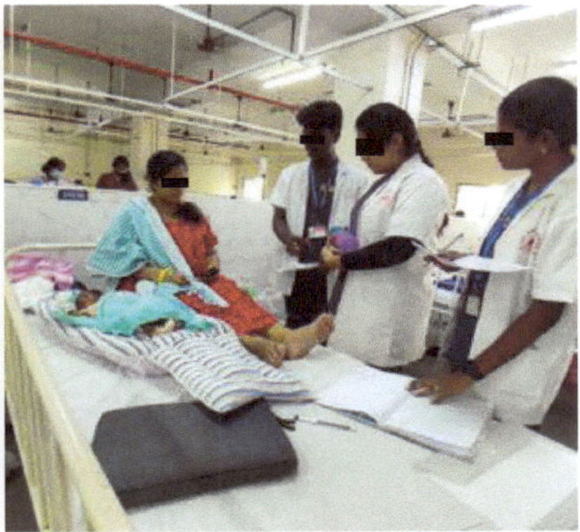

(b) **Postpartum Care**

Some of the conditions are:

- High-risk pregnancy
- Abortions/miscarriage
- Cancer
- Sexually Transmitted Diseases (STD)
- Uterine prolapse
- Polycystic Ovarian Syndrome (PCOS)
- Urinary incontinence
- Pelvic Inflammatory Disease (PID)

Role of Occupational Therapy in OBGYN

- **Prenatal education and preparation:** Occupational Therapists provide education and support to expectant mothers and their partners for proper body mechanics, exercise, and relaxation techniques. They help people prepare physically and emotionally for labor and delivery.
- **Labor and birth support:** Occupational Therapist provide emotional support, comfort measures during labor to help women cope with the physical and emotional challenges of childbirth.
- **Postpartum recovery:** Occupational Therapists provide postpartum care, including assessment of physical function, pain management strategies, and recommendations for adjusting daily activities during postpartum recovery. They can treat problems such as perineal discomfort, postural problems, and pelvic floor dysfunction.
- **Breastfeeding Support:** Occupational Therapists help new moms to breastfeed with guidance on proper positioning, latching techniques, and how to deal with breastfeeding difficulties or pain. They also recommend assistive devices such as breast pumps or nursing pads.
- **Postnatal depression and anxiety:** Occupational Therapists screen and support people with postnatal depression or anxiety. They offer strategies for managing stress, self-care routines and referrals to mental health professionals if needed.
- **Baby care and bonding:** Occupational Therapists train new parents in baby care techniques such as feeding, rocking, and fostering parent-child bonding. They also address any physical challenges or discomfort if parents experience while caring for their newborns.
- **Home safety and accessibility:** Occupational Therapists assess the home environment to ensure safety and accessbility for both the new mother and baby. They make recommendations about modifications or aids to support daily activities and reduce the risk of trauma.

- **Support for high-risk pregnancies:** For the high-risk pregnancies or complications, the Occupational Therapists work closely with the health care team to develop strategies to manage daily activities and maintain the best possible quality of life for the expectant mother.
- **Parenting Skills:** Occupational Therapists provide guidance on parenting skills such as infant and child development, sensory integration, and strategies for managing daily routines with a newborn or toddler.

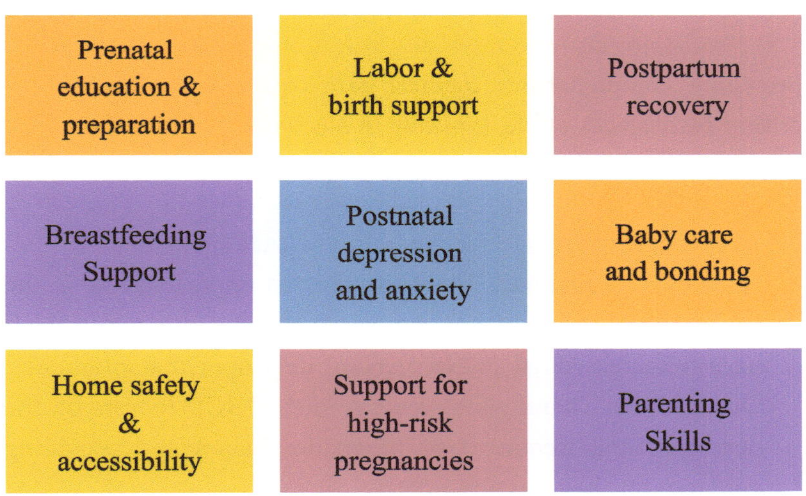

(Role of Occupational Therapy in OBGYN)

Summary

In general, OBGYN Occupational Therapists strive to improve the physical and emotional well-being of individuals during the prenatal, perinatal, and postpartum periods. They provide valuable support and training to help women and their families cope with the challenges and joys of pregnancy, childbirth, and early parenthood.

CHAPTER 5

NEONATOLOGY

Introduction

Neonatology focuses on the care of newborn infants, particularly those who are born prematurely, have low birth weights, or have medical conditions that require specialized attention.

Neonatologists are medical professionals who specialize in providing comprehensive medical care to newborns during the critical early stages of life, typically in Neonatal Intensive Care Unit (NICU) and other healthcare settings.

Role of Occupational Therapy in Neonatology

- Neonatal Occupational Therapists play an important role in the development of premature and fragile infants, as many of them have an increased risk of experiencing developmental difficulties.
- Occupational Therapy intervention in the NICU focuses on the developmental treatment of premature babies and providing guidance for their parents.
- Occupational Therapists who practice in neonatal setting have a comprehensive knowledge of the medical situation and unique developmental conditions that characterize the infant population.

The guidelines objectives include

- The goals support the clinical reasoning of Occupational Therapists with regard to promoting and providing high-risk infants with individualized care and encouraging their participation in relevant occupations. (e.g., sleeping, feeding, exploring, etc.).

- Working with individual families to negotiate their meaning of parenting and parent-infant shared occupations.
- Providing sensitive opportunities for parenting occupations to create more ordinary and positive experiences for parents and their infants within the neonatal unit.

Occupational Therapy intervention strategies

- Infant feeding techniques
- Positioning
- Parent engagement & support
- Early intervention
- Development support care
- Kangaroo care

Goals of Occupational Therapy

The Goal of Occupational Therapy services provided in neonatal settings is to support the growth of high-risk infants and their families. Occupational Therapists work with parents of high-risk infants to facilitate the infant's and parent's occupational roles, support the parent-infant relationship, and ensure a successful transition from hospital to home.

Continuous intervention and/or guidance offers ongoing opportunities to support the development of infant occupations around self-care, learning, and play as the infant grows older and is discharged from the unit by instructing parents in methods for encouraging and involving their infant in appropriate sensory and motor experiences.

Occupational Therapy Interventions

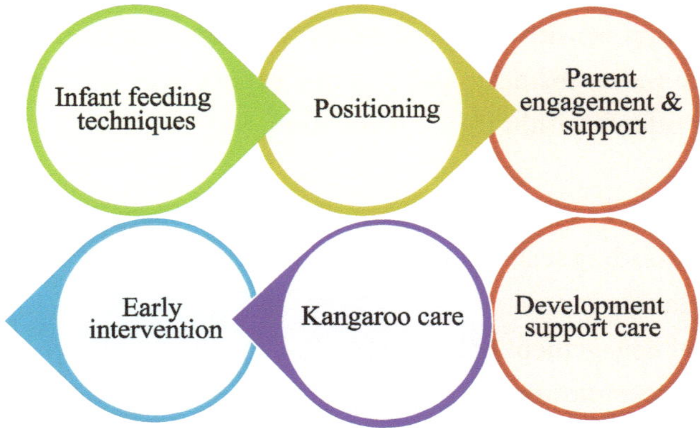

Summary

The overall role of Occupational Therapy in Neonatology is to promote optimal development, improve sensory-motor experiences. The ultimate goal is to facilitate the brain development through sensory motor stimulation. To facilitate the musculoskeletal function and reflex maturation.

CHAPTER 6

PAEDIATRICS

Introduction

A subspecialty of medicine called paediatrics is concerned with the health and wellbeing of new-born's, young children, adolescents, Paediatricians are medical professionals with specialized training in providing young patients with comprehensive healthcare that takes into account their physical, emotional, and developmental requirements.

Paediatric care is marked by a compassionate, family-centred approach. Paediatricians not only attend to the physical health of their patients but also consider the emotional and social aspects of their lives. They work closely with parents and caregivers to provide support and guidance throughout the child's development.

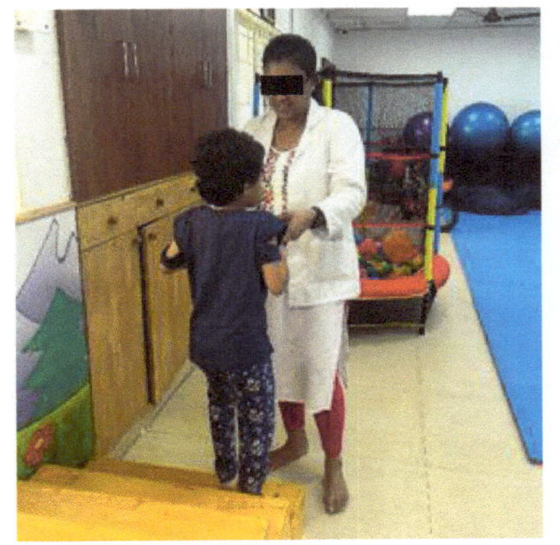

(a) Motor Planning Activity

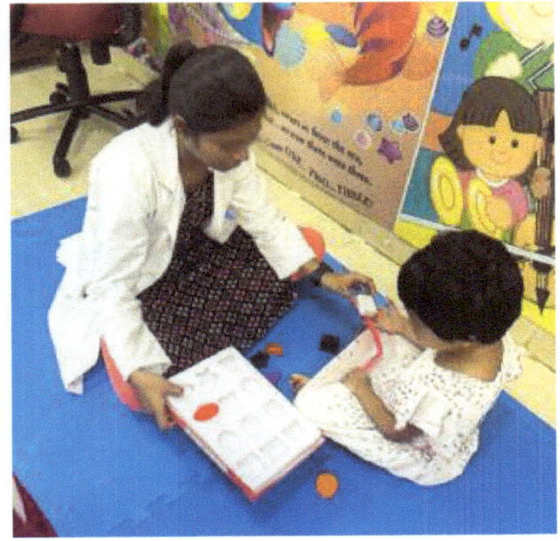

(b) Concept Training (Shape Board)

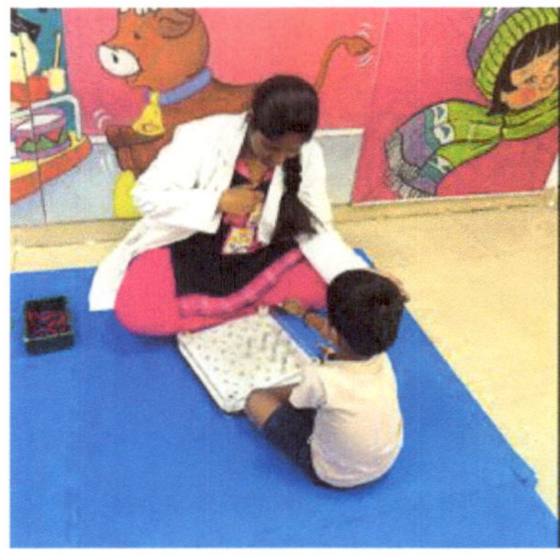

(c) **Task based activity**

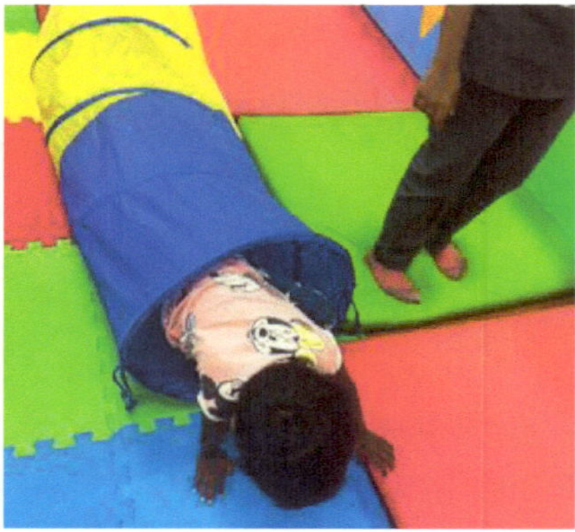

(d) **Crawling Activity**

Some Conditions are:

- Autism Spectrum Disorder
- ADD/ADHD
- Down's Syndrome
- Learning Disability
- Cerebral Palsy / Brain Injury
- Congenital Anomalies
- Developmental Delay
- Intellectual Disability
- Genetic Disorder
- Haemophilia
- Orthopaedic Injury or Surgery
- Cancer / Leukaemia

Role of Occupational Therapy for children

Occupational Therapists work with children who find it difficult to participate completely in regular daily life activities. These difficulties may be due to developmental delays, Attention Deficit Hyperactive Disorder, Autism, trauma, chromosomal problems, injuries, and many other conditions. An Occupational Therapist evaluates the child's areas of difficulty as well as their strengths and provides treatment directed to meet their requirements.

- **Developmental Milestones:** Occupational Therapists evaluate children's age-appropriate developmental milestones in areas including gross and fine motor skills, sensory processing, self care and social skills.
- **Early Intervention:** Occupational Therapists usually work with new-borns and young children who have developmental delays or conditions which affect their growth and development like Cerebral Palsy, Down syndrome, or Autism Spectrum Disorder.
- **Individualized Treatment Plans:** Occupational Therapists use to formulate individualized treatment plans tailored to the unique needs and strengths of each child. These plans aim to address specific challenges and promote developmental skills.
- **Sensory Processing:** Occupational Therapists assess and address sensory processing difficulties, helping children better regulate their responses to sensory stimuli, such as touch, sound, taste, vision and smell.
- **Gross Motor Skills:** Occupational Therapists help kids acquire the gross motor skills required for activities like stair climbing, cycling.
- **Fine-Motor Skills:** Fine motor abilities are necessary for tasks like clothing, writing, and using utensils, and Occupational Therapists work with children in developing these skills. Activities that enhance finger dexterity, hand strength, and eye - hand coordination are part of this.

- **Self-Care Skills:** Occupational Therapists help kids to develop the necessary self-care abilities, including clothing, feeding, using the restroom, and grooming. These skills are required to foster functional independence and enhance self-esteem.
- **Play and Social Skills:** By providing opportunities for kids to interact with their classmates and practice cooperation, communication, and problem-solving. Occupational Therapists promote the development of play skills and social interaction skills.
- **Environmental Adaptations:** Occupational Therapists provide recommendations for adapting a child's environment, whether at home, school, or in the community, to better accommodate their needs and promote participation.
- **School-Based Therapy:** Occupational Therapy plays a vital role in main stream school settings to promote the students academic performance and participation in classroom activities.
- **Multidisciplinary Approach:** Occupational Therapists work collaboratively with parents, teachers, medical professions, and other healthcare professionals to provide a comprehensive care for children. They also collaborate with Speech therapists, Physiotherapists, and Special educators to provide holistic support.

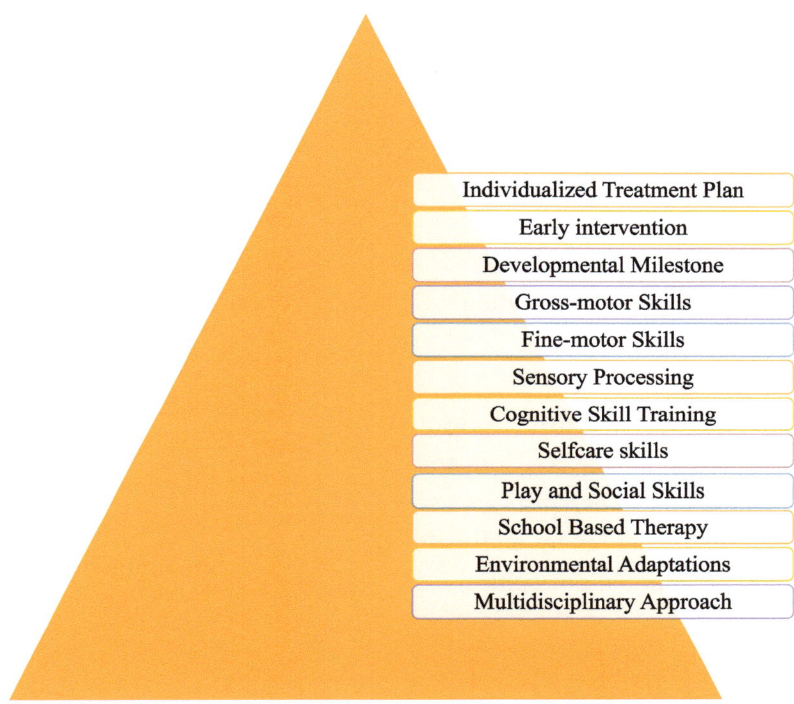

(Role of Occupational Therapy in Paediatrics)

Parental Involvement

Parents play a major role in child's development and parental participation in therapy is important for therapeutic outcomes. Parents provide valuable insights into the child's behaviour, emotions, development, and environment. The caregiver's active involvement in the intervention process is essential to the child's progress.

Occupational Therapy Service Offered:

- Sensory Integration Therapy
- Neuro Developmental Therapy
- Sensory-motor Training
- Cognitive skills training

- Oro-motor Skills Training
- Hand Function skills Training
- Handwriting Training
- Group Therapy
- Therapeutic Play
- Social skills Training
- Home Program
- Patient/Parent Education.

Summary

The goal of Paediatric Occupational Therapy is to enable child to participate in daily activities and reach their full potential. Paediatric Occupational Therapists are essential in enhancing the lives of kids and their families by addressing physical, sensory, cognitive, and social-emotional difficulties.

CHAPTER 7

SENSORY INTEGRATION THERAPY

Introduction

Sensory Integration Therapy is a therapeutic approach designed to help individuals who struggle with Sensory Processing Difficulties. Sensory Processing refers to how the nervous system receives, interprets, and responds to sensory information from the environment. This information includes input from the five senses (sight, hearing, taste, touch, and smell) as well as from the proprioceptive (body position) and vestibular (balance and spatial orientation) systems.

Some individuals, particularly those with Sensory Processing Disorders (SPD) or other developmental challenges such as Autism Spectrum Disorder (ASD), may have difficulty processing and integrating sensory information effectively. This can result in various challenges, including sensory over-responsivity, sensory under-responsivity, and difficulty with motor coordination and planning.

Sensory Integration Therapy aims to address these issues by providing structured, sensory-rich experiences to help individuals improve their ability to process and respond to sensory input appropriately.

Key principles of Sensory Integrative approach

- Just right challenge
- The adaptive response
- Active engagement
- Child-directed

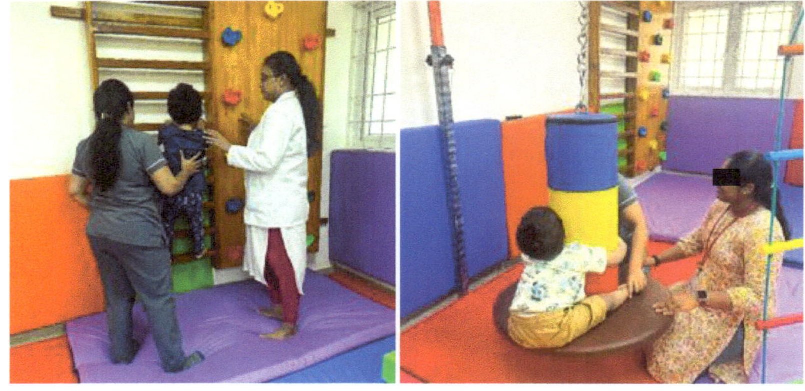

(a) Proprioceptive Activity **(b) Vestibular Activity**

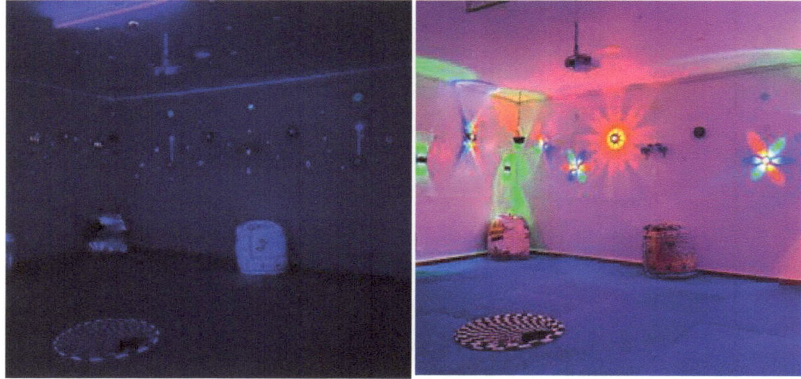

(c) (i) Multi Sensory Stimulation Room **(c) (ii) Multi Sensory Stimulation Room**

Areas of Practice

Sensory Processing is important in everyday activities, Children with SI difficulties have performance-related problems in all areas of daily life:

- Activities of Daily Living (ADL)
- Work, Play, Leisure
- Social participation

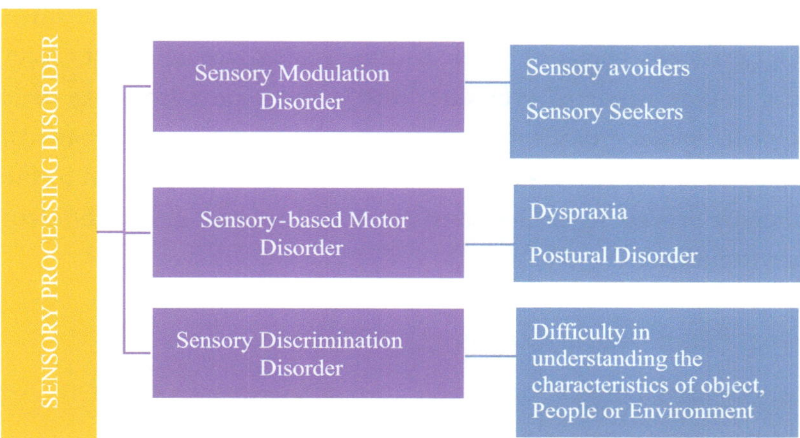

Sensory Integration Therapy offers

- A different perspective on understanding behaviour.
- Strategies to improve attention, motivation, communication, and interaction
- Physical and ecological housing
- Increasing self-esteem and confidence
- Snoezelen spaces, often referred to as multi-sensory environments, promote relaxation and social interaction.

Objective

The primary goal of Sensory Integration Therapy is to improve an individual's ability to process and respond to sensory information from their environment in a more adaptive and functional manner.

Target Population

- Sensory Processing Disorders (SPD)
- Autism Spectrum Disorder (ASD)
- Developmental Delays.

Sensory Integration Therapy should be provided by a qualified Occupational Therapist. Their treatment plans are tailored to meet the unique needs of everyone, with a focus on addressing their specific sensory challenges and goals. Collaboration with parents, caregivers, teachers, and other professionals is often integral to the therapy process to ensure consistency and support across different environments.

Benefits of Sensory Integration Therapy

- Improves sensory processing skills.
- Enhances motor coordination & motor planning.
- Increases self-regulation
- Improves overall functioning in daily life, learning, & social interactions

Summary

Sensory Integration Therapy is a therapeutic approach designed to help individuals with sensory processing difficulties improve their sensory processing abilities, adapt to sensory input, and enhance their overall quality of life through individualized, play-based, and structured interventions led by Occupational Therapist.

CHAPTER 8

ACUTE CARE

Introduction

The patients who are admitted for a short period to an acute care setup do have functional loss due to their critical condition at that time. These patients come across a sudden decline in their functional status and medical condition. Occupational Therapists help clients recover health and Quality of Life by facilitating involvement in meaningful occupations or work.

The primary purpose of Acute Care is to stabilize the patient's medical status and address life-threatening issues. Later the second most essential goal is to maintain or improve the Quality of Life by enhancing Functional Status and providing safety to facilitate early recovery and to reduce their hospitalization and to avoid physical, social and cognitive complications, these are the domains of Occupational Therapy.

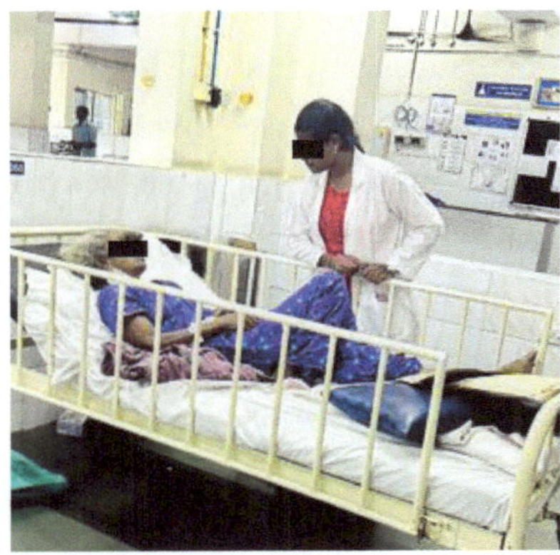

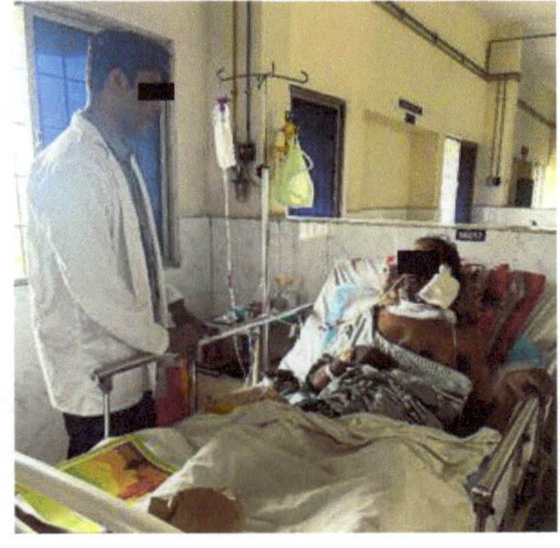

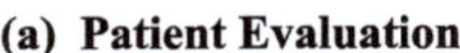

(a) Patient Evaluation

(b) Patient Health Education

Some of the Acute Care Conditions:

- Cardiac Disease
- Stroke
- Traumatic injuries

Role of Occupational Therapy in Acute Care

Occupational Therapy plays a crucial role in acute settings, such as hospitals and emergency departments, where patients are dealing with sudden and often serious medical conditions.

The primary goal of Occupational Therapy in acute care settings is to promote a patient's independence and functional ability while they are recovering from illness, injury, or surgery.

- **Assessment:** Occupational Therapists assess the patient's physical, cognitive, emotional, and psychosocial functioning to understand their unique needs and limitations. This assessment helps in developing individualized treatment plans.
- **Functional Evaluation:** Occupational Therapists evaluate a patient's ability to perform essential Basic Activities of Daily Living (BADLs) such as dressing, bathing, grooming, eating, and mobility. They also assess Instrumental Activities of Daily Living (IADLs) like cooking, cleaning, and managing finances.
- **Assistive Device Prescription:** Occupational Therapists recommend and provide training on the use of assistive devices such as wheelchairs, walkers, adaptive utensils, and splints to enhance the patient's independence and safety.
- **Patient and Caregiver education:** They educate patients and their families about strategies for managing daily activities, preventing complications, and making necessary adaptations to the home environment for a safe discharge.
- **Functional Mobility:** Occupational Therapists work on improving a patient's functional mobility and strength through therapeutic activities and techniques that target their specific needs. This can include helping patients regain balance and coordination.

- **Cognitive Rehabilitation:** In cases where patients have cognitive impairments due to conditions like stroke or traumatic brain injury, Occupational Therapists provide cognitive rehabilitation to improve memory, problem-solving, and decision-making skills.
- **Pain Management:** Occupational Therapists use techniques like positioning, therapeutic modalities, and activity modification to help manage pain and discomfort in acute care settings.
- **Psychosocial Support:** They offer emotional support and coping strategies to help patients and their families adjust to the challenges of acute illness or injury.
- **Adaptive Strategies:** Occupational Therapists teach patients adaptive strategies to compensate for any permanent or long-term functional limitations, enabling them to participate in meaningful activities.
- **Ergonomic Modifications:** Occupational Therapists assess the ergonomic aspects of a patient's work or home environment to prevent future injuries or improve productivity. Occupational Therapist provide Work Simplification, Energy Conservation and Joint Protection Techniques.
- **Discharge Planning:** Occupational Therapists collaborate with the healthcare team to plan for a safe and smooth discharge. They recommend home modifications, adaptive equipment, or home health services to ensure a successful transition from the hospital.
- **Multidisciplinary Collaboration:** They work closely with other healthcare professionals, including Physicians, Physical Therapists, Speech Therapists, and Social Workers, to provide holistic care to the patient.

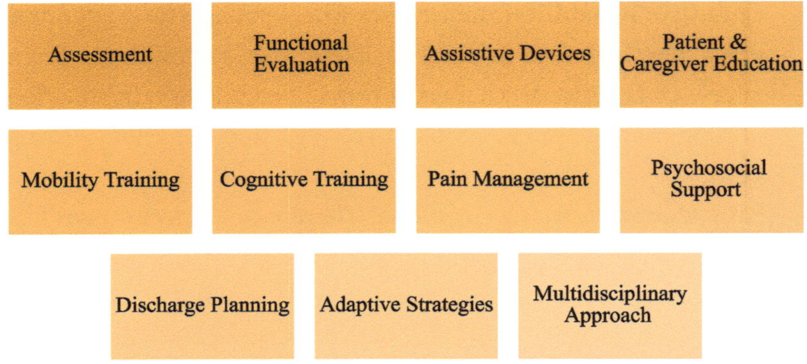

(Role of Occupational Therapy in Acute Care)

Summary

In acute care settings, Occupational Therapists play a critical role in facilitating the early recovery and the overall well-being and functional independence of patients, helping them regain their abilities and ultimately transition back to their home and community environments.

CHAPTER 9

ORTHOPAEDICS

Introduction

Occupational Therapy have a significant positive impact on patients healing from musculoskeletal disorders or accidents where adequate movement has been restricted. Through examination, planning, execution, and evaluation of the management of the injury or condition. Occupational Therapy aims to improve the balance and functionality of the patient's musculoskeletal system.

In orthopaedics, an Occupational Therapist's help patients deal with and get rid of the restrictions brought on by their illness or disability. It is intended that with the support of the Occupational Therapist, the patient would be able to improve the quality of their life by assisting them in working and living independently and helping to improve their overall health.

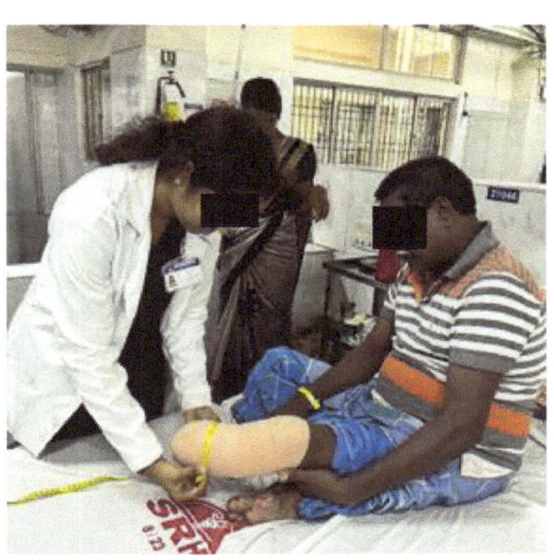

(a) Stump Evaluation

Their role is to encourage the patient to take part in routine activities including getting dressed and taking off their clothes, finding work or going to school or training, and engaging in social and leisure activities. The Occupational Therapist suggest and provide training on the use of Wheelchair and other Mobility Aids. The Occupational Therapist also evaluates the patient's home and work evironment suggesting modification to fit for their needs.

The common conditions are:

- Lower back pain
- Cumulative trauma disorder
- Ligament Injury
- Fracture
- Bursitis
- Arthritis
- Osteoporosis
- Osteomyelitis
- Deformations of the spine
- Congenital malformations
- Bone tumour's
- Diabetic foot ulcer
- Amputation
- Perthes disease of calves

Role of Occupational Therapy in Orthopaedics

- **Screening and Evaluation:** Occupational Therapists start by evaluating a person's physical and functional capacities. They evaluate the impact of the orthopaedic condition on daily activities and functional independence.
- **Customized Treatment Plans:** Based on the assessment, Occupational Therapists create tailored treatment plans to address the patient's specific requirements and goals.

- **Pain Management:** Orthopaedic conditions are more painful. Occupational Therapists work on strategies to manage pain, which can include various methods such as Jacobson's Muscle Relaxation Techniques, Joint Protection Techniques and Body Mechanics Education.
- **Range of Motion and Strength Training:** Occupational Therapists help patients through activities meant to improve joint range of motion and muscle strength, enabling better mobility and stability.
- **Activities of Daily Living (ADL) Training:** ADLs are fundamental task which the people perform daily, such as dressing, bathing, grooming, and cooking. Occupational Therapist teach patients techniques and adaptations to perform these activities independently or with less difficulty.
- **Assistive Devices and Adaptive Equipment:** Occupational Therapist recommend and teaches Energy Conservation, Work Simplification and adaptive strategies to perform these daily activities independently.
- **Environmental Modifications:** Occupational Therapist assess the patient's home and workplace and suggest modifications or adaptations to ensure safety and accessibility. This could include installing grab bars, ramps, or ergonomic furniture.
- **Psychosocial Support:** Injuries and treatment will cause a negative impact on one's mental health. By providing emotional support and coping strategies, Occupational Therapists assist patients in managing the psychological components of their condition.
- **Work and Leisure Activities:** Occupational Therapist work with patients to help them return to work and engage in leisure activities safely. This may involve job site evaluations, ergonomic recommendations, and leisure activity modifications.

- **Patient Education:** Occupational Therapist educate patients about their condition, recovery process, and strategies to prevent future injuries. This includes teaching proper body mechanics and ergonomics.
- **Home Programs:** Patients are often given home programs to continue their rehabilitation independently, ensuring continued progress.
- **Follow-Up and Monitoring:** Occupational Therapists follow up with patients to track progress, make adjustments to treatment plans, and address any new challenges that may arise during recovery.

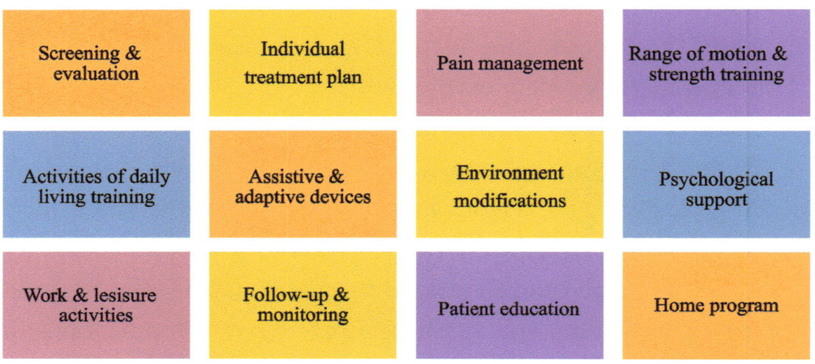

(Role of Occupational Therapy in Orthopaedics)

Summary

In orthopaedics, the goal of Occupational Therapy is to maximize a patient's functional independence, improve their overall quality of life, and facilitate a safe return to their daily activities, work, and hobbies. The specific interventions and techniques used by Occupational Therapists vary depending on the individual's orthopaedic condition and their unique needs and goals.

Chapter 10

NEUROLOGY

Introduction

Neurological disorders can affect various aspects of a person's life including motor skills, cognitive function, sensory perception and Psychosocial well-being. Neurological Occupational Therapy is a specialty that focuses on helping people with neurological diseases or disorders to become more independent, in Activites of Daily Living and to improve Quality Of Life.

Occupational Therapists have extensive experience working with clients with brain injury or other neurological diagnoses, as well as physical, mental health or social problems. They offer a client-centered service that includes individualized assessment and adult rehabilitation aimed at optimizing the client's functional independence and functional abilities.

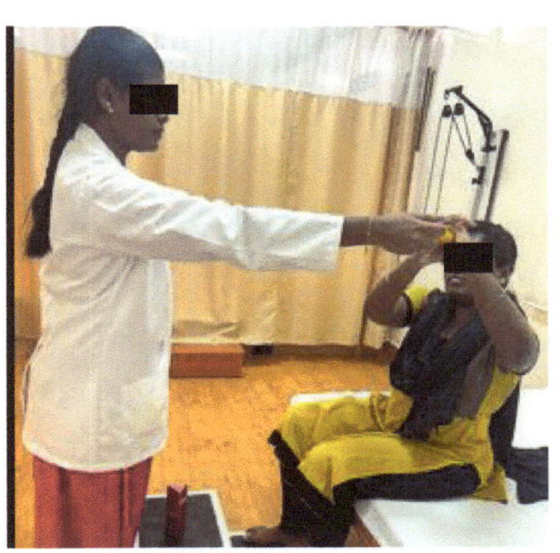

(a) Neuro Occupational Therapy Intervention

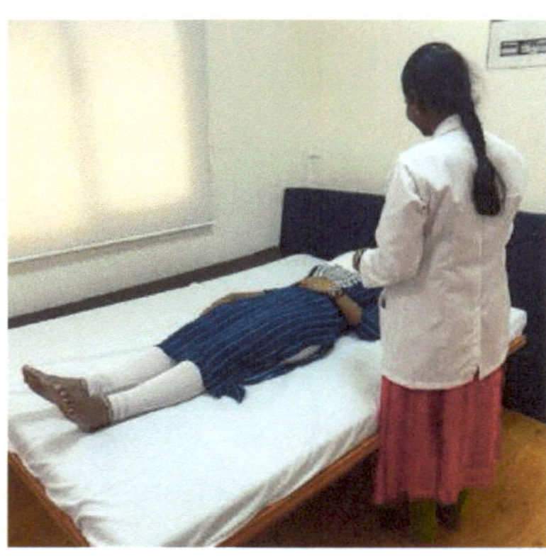

(b) Occupational Therapy Education - Bed Positioning

Aims of Occupational Therapy in Neurology

- To maximize patient's functional independence
- To promote patient's participation in Occupational Performance
- To promote Quality of Life (QoL)
- To facilitate Community Re-integration

Occupational Therapists specialize in treating the following Neurological conditions

- Cerebral Vascular Accident (CVA)
- Brain Injury / Brain tumour
- Multiple Sclerosis (MS)
- Spinal Cord Injury (SCI)
- Parkinson's Disease (PD)
- Muscular Dystrophy (MD)
- Myasthenia Gravis
- Peripheral Nerve Injury
- Poliomyelitis and Post Polio Syndrome
- Guillain Barre Syndrome (GBS)
- Motor Neuron Disease (MND)
- Vestibular Disorders

Assessment

Assessment begins with observation of the patient performing various tasks and a clinical interview that includes open-ended questions about medical and work history, physical and social environment, and standardized assessments such as Sensorimotor, perceptual, cognitive, and executive function tests.

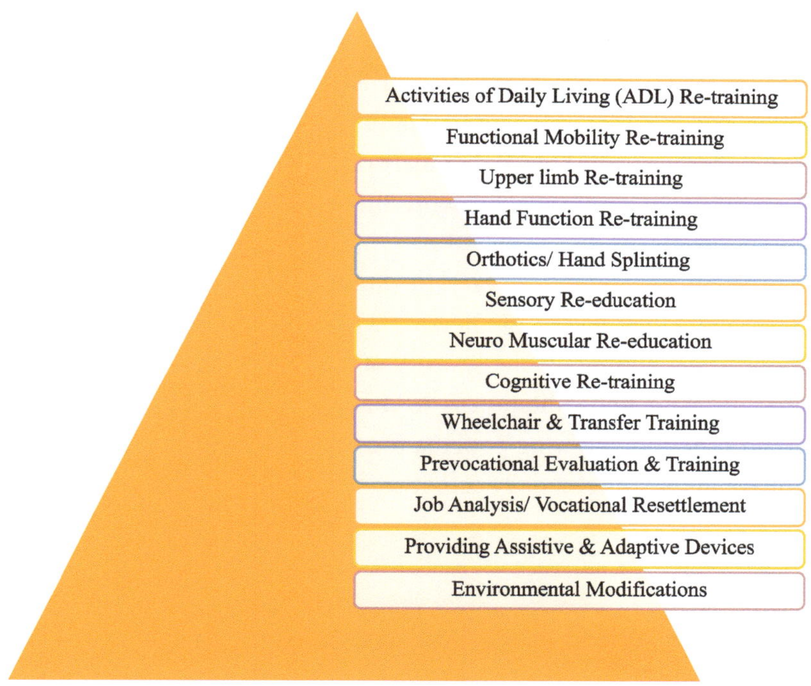

(Occupational Therapy Interventions in Neurology)

Summary

Occupational Therapists collaborate closely with other healthcare professionals, including Physiotherapist, Speech-Language pathologists, and neurologists, to provide holistic care. Occupational Therapy interventions aim to maximize a person's functional independence, promote quality of life, and adapt to changing needs as individuals progress in their recovery or manage their conditions over time.

Chapter 11

HAND REHABILITATION

Hand Rehabilitation is a specialized form of Occupational Therapy that focuses on improving the function and mobility of the Hand, Wrist, and Upper Extremity. It is often required for individuals who have experienced Hand injuries, undergone Hand surgery, or conditions that affect their Hand function. The goal of Hand Rehabilitation is to help individuals regain strength, flexibility, and dexterity in their Hands, allowing them to perform daily activities and tasks effectively.

Hand Rehabilitation vary in duration, with some individuals requiring a few weeks of therapy, while others may need several months, depending on the severity of their condition. The ultimate goal of Hand Rehabilitation is to maximize recovery and improve Hand function, allowing patients to regain their independence and engage in meaningful daily activities.

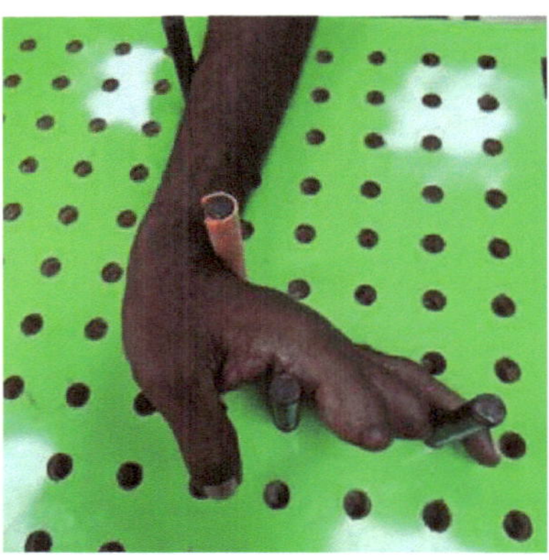

a) Occupational Therapy Intervention - Stretch Board

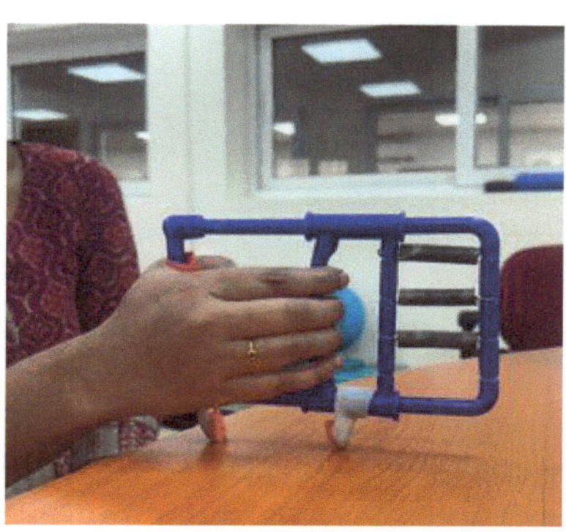

(b) Occupational Therapy Intervention - Hand Strengthening

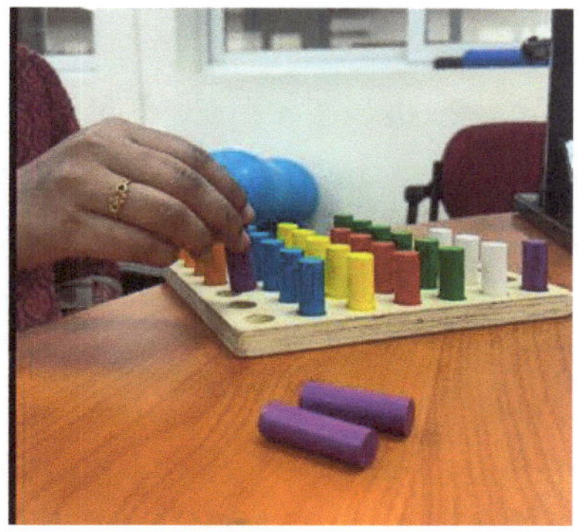

(c) Occupational Therapy Intervention - Hand Function Activity

Conditions of Hand Rehabilitation

- Fracture
- Tendon injuries
- Nerve injuries
- Arthritis
- Amputation
- Dupuytren's Contracture
- Burns
- Stroke
- Spinal Cord Injury
- Rheumatoid Arthritis

- Cubital Tunnel Syndrome
- Trigger Finger
- Work-related Injuries
- Congenital Conditions

Role of Occupational Therapy

- **Assessment:**
    - Hand Rehabilitation begins with a thorough assessment to determine the specific impairments and limitations in Hand function. This includes evaluating range of motion, strength, sensation, coordination and fine motor skills.
- **Treatment Plan:**
    - Based on the assessment, a individualized treatment plan is developed to address the individual's unique needs and goals. The plan may include activities, therapeutic modalities, and other interventions.
- **Activities:**
    - Occupational Therapists teach patients a range of activities and provide joint mobility based activities. These activities are often tailored to the individual's condition and may include grip strength activities, finger dexterity activities, and more.
- **Splinting and Orthotics:**
    - Occupational Therapists design and provide customized splints or orthotic devices to support the Hand during the healing process and to prevent deformities.
- **Pain and Odema Management:**
    - Occupational Therapist provide paraffin wax, fluidotherapy and techniques to control odema.
- **Functional Training:**
    - Occupational Therapists work on improving an individual's ability to perform daily activities, such as dressing, eating, writing, and using tools or instruments.

- **Education:**
  - Patients are educated about their condition, preventive measures, and strategies for self-care at home.
- **Scar Management:**
  - If the patient has surgical scars, therapists may provide guidance on managing and massaging scars to minimize their impact on Hand function.
- **Adaptive Techniques:**
  - Learning adaptive techniques and tools that can make tasks easier for individuals with Hand limitations.
- **Progress Monitoring:**
  - Progress is monitored throughout the Rehabilitation process, and the treatment plan is adjusted as needed.

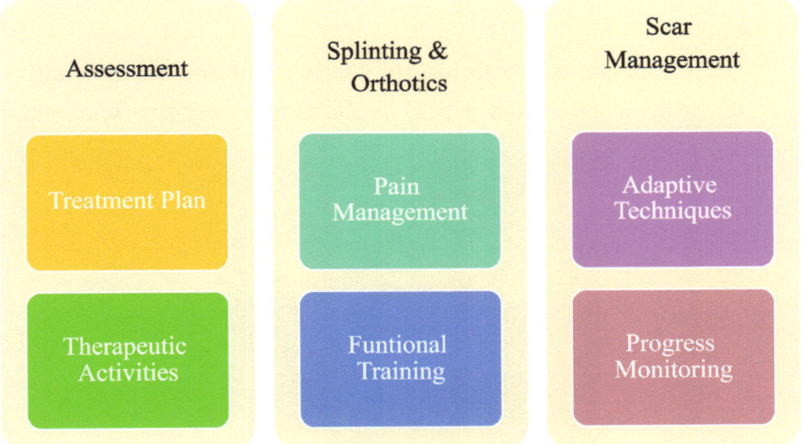

Summary

Hand Rehabilitation is often provided by Occupational Therapists with specialized training in Hand and Upper Extremity Rehabilitation. The duration and intensity of Hand Rehabilitation vary depending on the individual's condition and goals.

CHAPTER 12

HAND SPLINTING

Introduction

Occupational Therapists work closely with surgeons in order to provide the best outcomes for their patients. Occupational Therapist brings an added dimension to this specialty area. We use an Occupation-Based and Client-Centred Approach that identifies the participation needs (what he or she wants in their daily life that is fulfilling, necessary and meaningful). Occupational Therapist emphasize the performance of desired activities as the primary goal of therapy.

Hand and hand functions, are such a vital and demonstrative part of the body which has critical implication on occupational tasks.

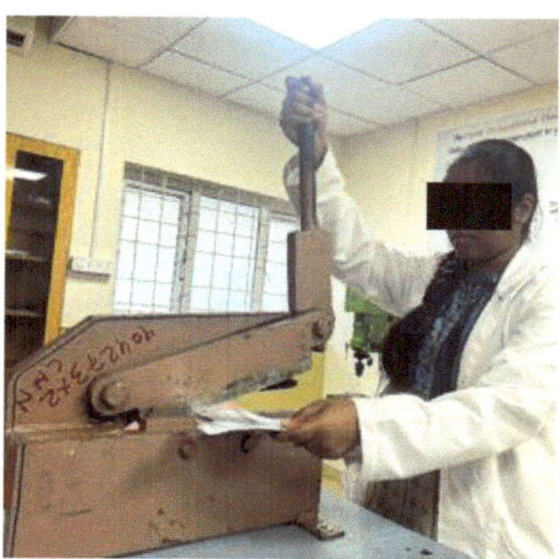

(a) Hand Splinting process - Aluminium Sheet Cutting

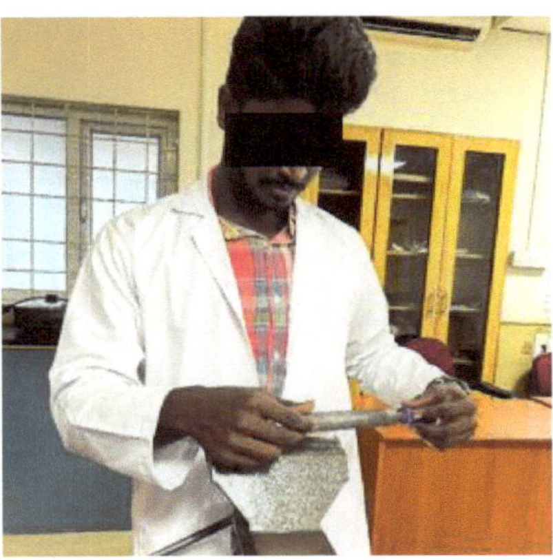

(b) Hand Splinting process - Filing

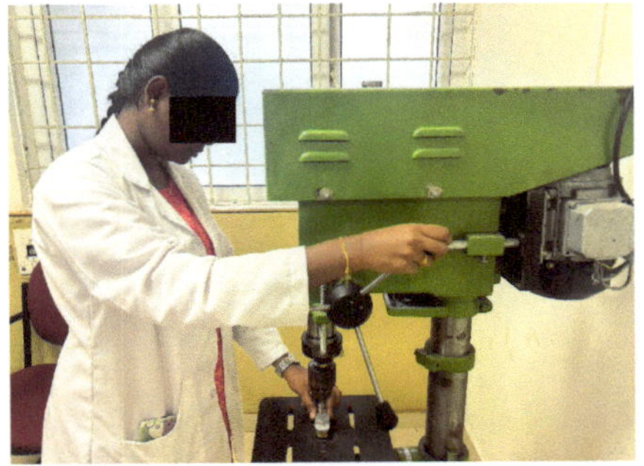

(c) Hand Splinting process - Drilling

How Occupational Therapist are Different in Hand Splinting Interventions

Occupational Therapists design splints based on various rehabilitation strategies by selecting the appropriate splint design based on the following.

- Diagnosis and prognosis
- Medical Complications
- Occupational Performance
- Social environment
- Client's comfort

- Caregivers comfort
- Age and gender of the person

Occupational Therapist Role

- Occupational Therapy is the health care profession that aims to restore a patient's functional capacity.
- Limit the progression of the disease or prevent upper limb dysfunction.
- To help patients resume their everyday task at home and at work and their recreational activities.
- Occupational Therapist make customized splints for the specific needs of each person or may use pre- fabricated splints.
- Providing Patient Education.
- Performs a checkout to verify its fit and comfort to assure that the patient understands its use and care.

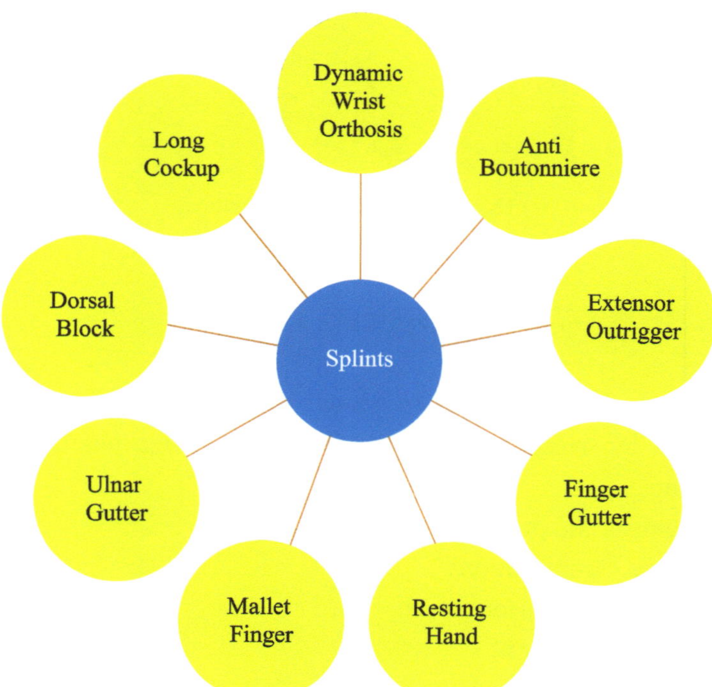

Summary

Occupational Therapists play a crucial role in Hand Rehabilitation, working closely with surgeons to enhance patients' outcomes. They prioritize a client-centred approach, focusing on restoring a patient's ability to perform daily activities. Occupational Therapists aim to limit the progression of hand pathologies, prevent upper limb dysfunction, and help patients resume their everyday tasks. They create customized splints or use pre-fabricated ones, provide patient education, and ensure proper fit and comfort. Splinting benefit individuals with different conditions like arthritis, stroke, and spinal cord injuries.

CHAPTER 13

MENTAL HEALTH

Introduction

Emotional, psychological, and social well-being are all included in the concept of mental health, which is vital to human wellbeing. It describes a person's capacity to handle stress, uphold wholesome relationships, and make wise judgments as well as their cognitive and emotional resilience. A person's quality of life is greatly influenced by their mental health, which is a critical aspect of overall health.

Conversely, poor mental health, often referred to as mental illness or psychological disorders, can have a profound impact on a person's life. Conditions like Depression, Anxiety, Bipolar disorder, Schizophrenia, and others can affect thoughts, emotions, and behaviours. Fortunately, many of these conditions are treatable with the right care and support.

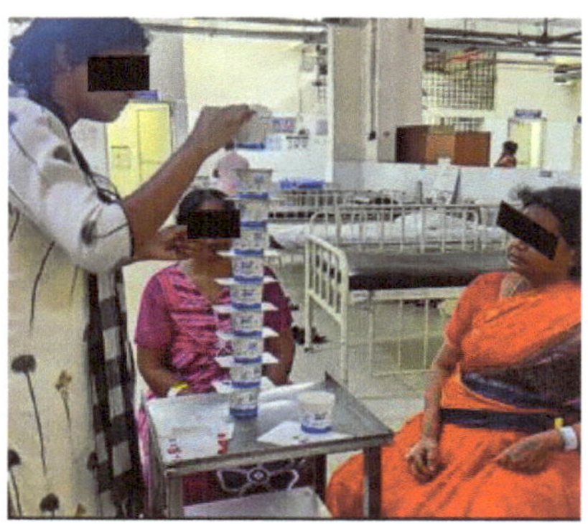

(a) Recreational Activity – Group Therapy (Cup Stacking)

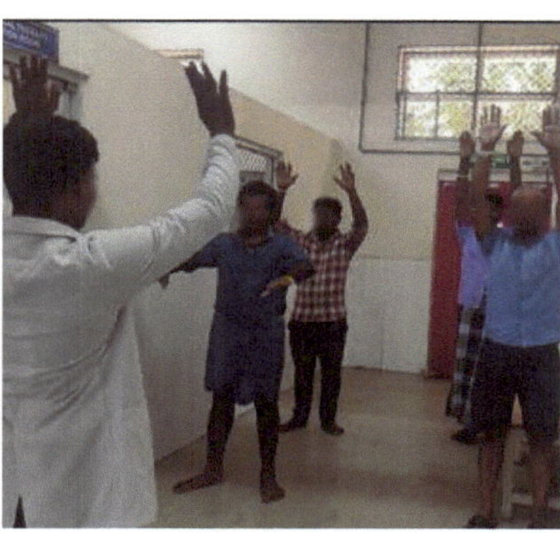

(b) Group Therapy

Need of Occupational Therapy?

Mentally healthy person leads a balanced and satisfying life, their energies divided among work, leisure, self-care, and care of others. They manage the conflicting demands of instincts (such as drives for sex and self- preservation), conscience (internalized moral rules and standards of behaviour), significant other people in their life, and the real external world.

People who have mental health problems do not just have trouble controlling their feelings and thoughts but also have difficulty with doing everyday activities and things that all of us take for granted.

Occupational Therapists are concerned with how people carry out their daily life activities and how well they perform the activities. Occupational Therapy uses carefully selected purposeful activities to help mentally ill individuals, families and communities learning new skills, maintain successful and adaptive habits, explore their feelings and interest and control their own life and destiny.

The purpose is to assess the patient's potential and interest in various kinds of work, and to help them, through discussion to select an area for further training.

Goals:

- Promote Positive Thoughts
- To Regulate the Mood
- Activities of Daily Living (ADL)
- Self responsibility
- Self awareness
- Self esteem
- Vocational resettlement
- Work adjustment
- Time management
- Leisure planning skills

Conditions:

- Schizophrenia
- Mood Disorder
- Anxiety Disorder
- Substance Use Disorder
- Psychosomatic Disorder
- Somatoform Disorder
- Sexual Disorder
- Eating Disorder
- Sleeping Disorder
- Obsessive Compulsive Disorder
- Dementia /Geriatric conditions

Occupational Therapy Intervention:

- Behavioural Modification
- ADL and Activity Scheduling
- Social Skills Training
- Vocational Training
- Job Analysis
- Leisure enhancement (Craft, Hobbies, Arts, games)
- Psychosocial Skill Training
- Assertiveness Training
- Anger/ Anxiety Management
- Stress Management

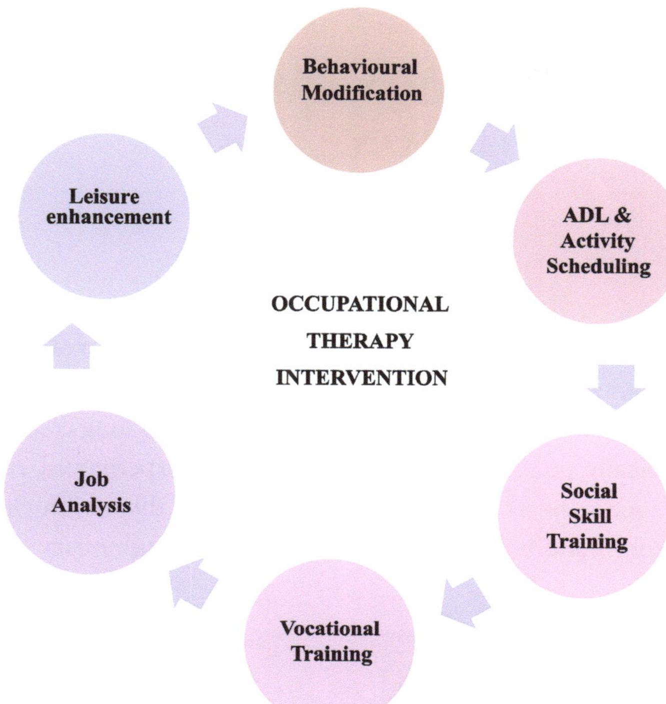

Services In

- Mental health setups
- Sheltered workshops
- Day care centres
- Half way homes
- Community - Based Mental Health Centres
- Governmental organizations
- NGOs

Summary

Occupational Therapy in mental health focuses on fulfilling lives by improving their mental well-being, promoting self-care and independence, and enhancing their overall quality of life.

Chapter 14

CARDIO-PULMONARY REHABILITATION

What is Cardio-pulmonary Rehabilitation?

Cardiopulmonary Rehabilitation is a structured program of exercise, education, and support designed to improve the physical and psychological well-being of individuals with heart or lung conditions. It is typically prescribed for people who have experienced cardiac events such as heart attacks, or heart surgery, or those with chronic respiratory conditions like chronic obstructive pulmonary disease (COPD).

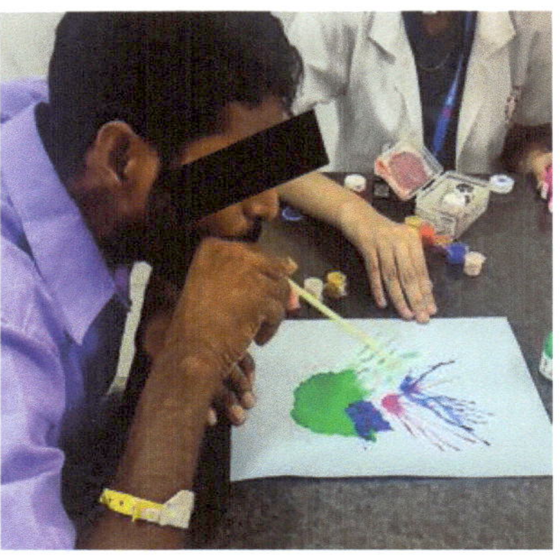

Breathing Activity - Blow Painting

Cardio-pulmonary conditions intervened by Occupational Therapists

- Systemic Hypertension
- Atrial Fibrillation

- Coronary Artery Disease (CAD)
- Congestive Cardiac Failure (CCF)
- Myocardial Infarction (MI)
- Angina Pectoris
- Congenital Heart Disease (CHD)
- Chronic Obstructive Pulmonary Disease (COPD)
- Asthma
- Chronic Bronchitis
- Lung Emphysema & Cancer

Phases of Occupational Therapy Rehabilitation

- **Phase I**- The acute phase focuses on ICU Care by monitoring vitals and providing Client and caregiver education.
- **Phase II**- The sub-acute setting focuses on Early Intervention and Complication Prevention
- **Phase III**- Rehab Facility or Outpatient Unit focuses on Intensive Therapy and Education
- **Phase IV**- Community Rehabilitation focuses on maintaining Optimal Health and Functional Independence

Role of Occupational Therapy in Cardio-Pulmonary Rehabilitation

Occupational Therapists support patients using environmental and contextual factors that can lead to healthy behaviours outside of the clinical setting Occupational Therapy plays a crucial role in Cardio-Pulmonary Rehabilitation by addressing the functional limitations and helping individuals regain independence and improving their quality of life following cardiovascular and pulmonary conditions and surgeries.

Here are the key roles and contributions of Occupational Therapy in Cardio-Pulmonary Rehabilitation:

Screening
&
Evaluation
Activity
Tolerance
M.E.T based
activity
Energy
Conservation
& Work
Simplification
ADL
Training
Home
Modification
&
Assistive
Devices
Psychosocial
Support
Activity
Scheduling
Education
& Lifestyle
Management
Work &
Leisure
Activity
Multi
disciplinary
Approach
Role of
OT

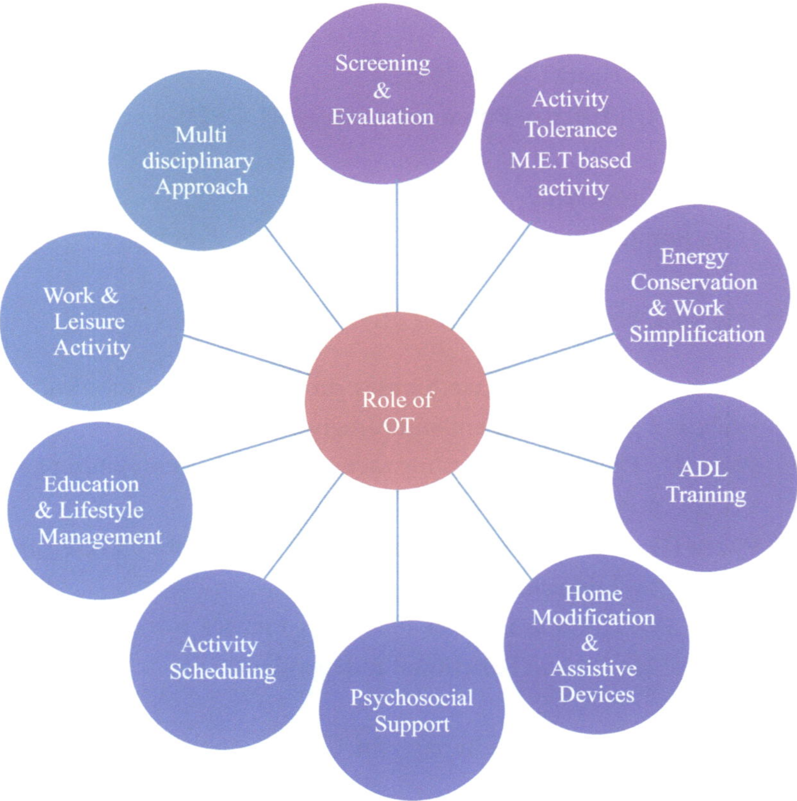

- **Screening and Evaluation:** Occupational Therapists assess the individual's physical, cognitive, and psychosocial functioning to identify their specific needs and limitations.
- **Activity Tolerance and Endurance Training:** Occupational Therapists develop personalized activity plans to improve cardiovascular endurance and overall strength. Occupational Therapist uses various techniques to increase tolerance for daily activities.

- **Energy Conservation and Work Simplification:** Occupational Therapists provide strategies to conserve energy during daily tasks, reducing fatigue and improving stamina. They teach individuals how to prioritize activities and plan their daily routines effectively.
- **ADL Training:** Occupational Therapists assist in relearning or adapting activities of daily living such as dressing, bathing, and meal preparation, to accommodate any physical limitations. They help individuals regain independence in these essential tasks.
- **Home Modification and Assistive Devices:** Occupational Therapists recommend home modifications and assistive devices to improve safety and accessibility. They ensure that the individual's home environment supports their recovery.
- **Psychosocial Support:** Occupational Therapists address the emotional and psychological aspects of recovery. They provide support and coping strategies for anxiety, depression, and the psychological impact of cardiac or pulmonary conditions.
- **Medication management:** Occupational Therapists educate individuals about medication management, ensuring they understand their prescriptions, dosages, and potential side effects.
- **Education and Lifestyle Management:** Occupational Therapists educate individuals about risk factors, lifestyle modifications, and preventive measures to reduce the risk of recurrent cardiac or pulmonary events.
- **Work and Leisure Activity:** Occupational Therapists work with individuals to help them return to or modify their work and leisure activities, ensuring they can engage in meaningful occupations.
- **Multidisciplinary Approach:** Occupational Therapists collaborate with other healthcare professionals, including physical therapists, physicians, nurses, and dietitians, to provide comprehensive care and ensure a holistic approach to rehabilitation

Self-Monitoring Technique

Occupational Therapists teach patients how to monitor their body's response to activity and warning signs that may need rest or medical attention.

Self-monitoring is an essential component of cardiac and pulmonary rehabilitation programs, helping individuals with heart and lung conditions track their progress, manage symptoms, and make informed decisions about their health.

Here's how self-monitoring can be applied in the context of cardiac and pulmonary rehabilitation

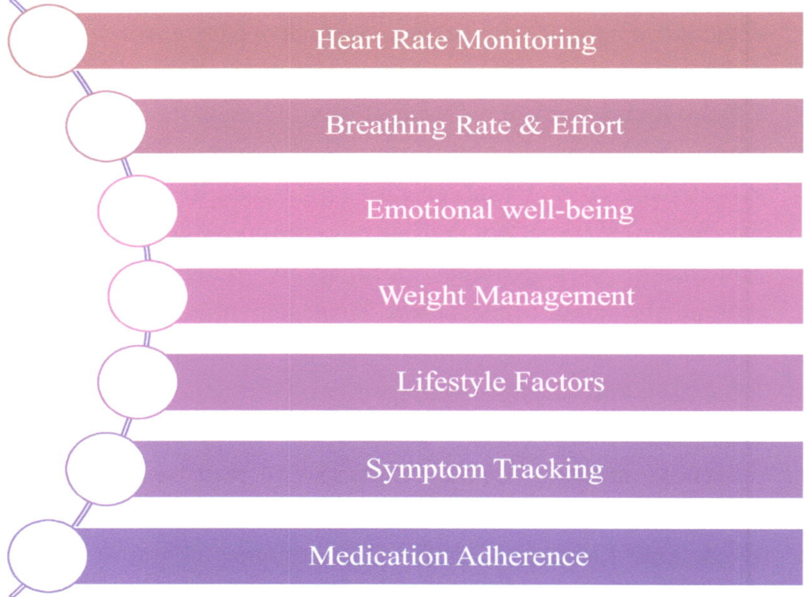

Summary

Occupational Therapists work as part of a multidisciplinary healthcare team to provide comprehensive care for individuals with cardiopulmonary conditions. Their goal is to enhance the overall quality of life for these individuals by helping them achieve and maintain the highest level of independence possible while managing their heart and lung conditions effectively.

Chapter 15

ENT - EAR, NOSE AND THROAT

Introduction

ENT (Ear, Nose, and Throat) specialists, also known as otolaryngologists, plays a vital role in treating a wide range of conditions and disorders related to the head and neck.

ENT specialists' expertise is essential in helping patients manage these conditions, improve their health, and enhance their overall well-being.

Occupational Therapy Role in ENT:

- **Swallowing and Feeding Disorders:** They assess and provide interventions to improve oral motor skills and functions. This is particularly important for individuals with conditions like dysphagia, which may result from surgeries or throat issues.
- **Adaptive Equipment and Assistive Technology:** Occupational Therapists may recommend and train individuals on the use of adaptive equipment and assistive technology to improve daily living and communication.
- **Tinnitus Management:** Tinnitus is a common symptom in ENT patients. Occupational Therapists can provide counselling and strategies for managing tinnitus-related stress and anxiety, as well as techniques like sound Therapy to help patients cope with the noise.
- **Psychosocial Support:** ENT conditions, particularly those involving head and neck surgeries or cancer, can have a significant impact on a person's psychosocial well-being. Occupational Therapists provide emotional support, coping strategies, and stress management techniques to help patients and their families navigate these challenges.

- **Rehabilitation Post-Surgery:** After ENT surgeries, Occupational Therapists assist with postsurgical rehabilitation, including scar management, pain management, and activities to regain strength and mobility in the head and neck region.
- **Environmental Modifications:** Occupational Therapists recommend and implement environmental modifications in the home or workplace to support individuals with hearing or communication difficulties, such as improving lighting, reducing background noise, or installing visual alerts for doorbells and phones.

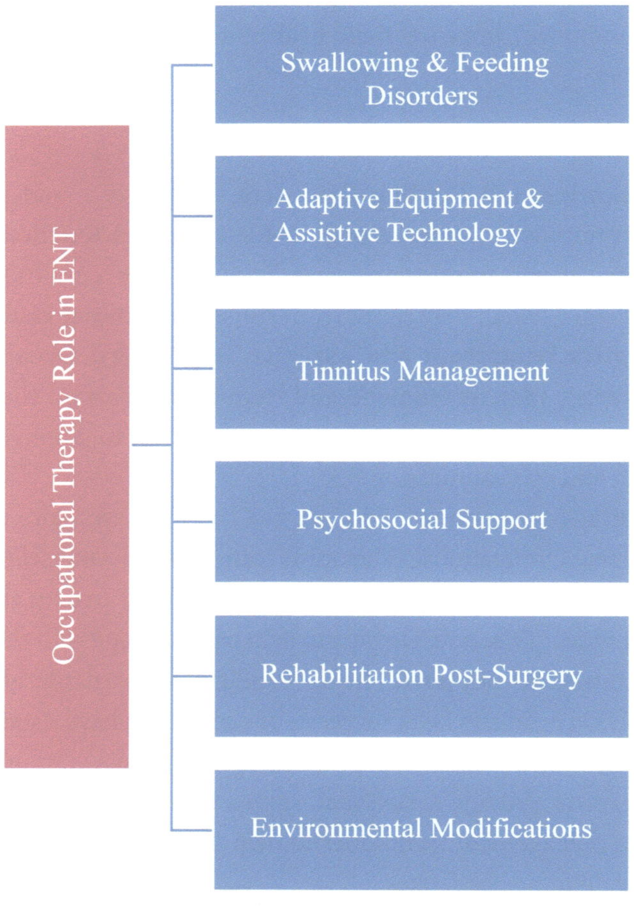

Summary

Occupational Therapy services in the ENT setting depends on the specific condition, the healthcare team's composition. Collaborative care among ENT specialists, speech-language pathologists, and Occupational Therapists provides comprehensive support for patients with ear, nose, and throat conditions.

Chapter 16

BURNS REHABILITATION

Introduction

Restoration of functional independence is the goal of burn rehabilitation. Functional restoration includes all aspects of human life such as strength, ROM, mobility and self-care, reintegration into family and community, adaptive psychosocial responses, and self-determination.

Goals of Rehabilitation

Acute Phase

- Provide cognitive reorientation and psychological support.
- Reduce oedema.
- Prevent loss of joint and skin mobility.
- Prevent loss of strength and activity tolerance.
- Promote occupational performance, such as independence in self-care skills.
- Provide patient and caregiver education.

Surgical and Postoperative Phase

- Promote cognitive awareness by providing orientation activities when necessary and continuing psychological support.
- Protect and preserve graft and donor sites by fabricating customized splints and establishing positioning techniques that support the surgeon's postoperative care orders.
- Prevent muscular atrophy and loss of activity tolerance.
- Increase independence in self-care by teaching alternative techniques and providing adaptive equipment as needed.

- Educate and reassure the patient and family members regarding this phase of recovery.

Rehabilitation Phase

- Improve joint mobility and reduce contractures by using correct positioning, sustained passive stretching exercises, and splinting as needed.
- Restore muscle strength, coordination, and activity tolerance.
- Initiate compression therapy and scar management.
- Promote independent self-care skills or the ability to direct others to assist when needed, including appropriate positioning, exercise, and skin care. Provide instruction and opportunities to practice Instrumental Activities of Daily living (IADLs), including vocational and home-care activities.
- Guide the implementation of a post-discharge plan that supports resumption of school, work, social, and leisure occupations.

Occupational Therapy Intervention

Acute Phase

- Client Education
- Preventive Positioning
- Splinting

Surgical and Postoperative Phase

- Positioning and Postoperative Splinting
- Therapeutic Exercise and Activity
- Activities of Daily Living training

Rehabilitation Phase

- Skin Conditioning and Scar Massage
- Compression Therapy
- Therapeutic Exercise and Activity

- Oedema Management
- Activities of Daily Living training
- Splinting
- Psychological Adjustment
- Community re-integration

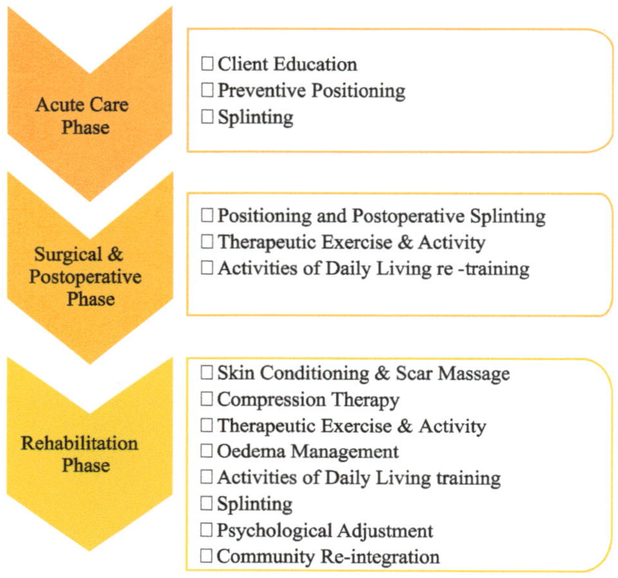

Summary

Occupational Therapy plays a crucial role in burns rehabilitation by helping individuals who have suffered from burn injuries regain their independence, functionality, and quality of life. Burn injuries can result in physical, emotional, and psychosocial challenges, and Occupational Therapists are trained to address these issues.

Chapter 17

VISUAL REHABILITATION

Visual impairment is defined as the loss of or deficits in visual function due to pathology or processing problems in one or more components of the visual system that limits the individual's ability to engage in and participate in daily occupations.

Visual Rehabilitation is a comprehensive and collaborative approach to helping individuals with visual impairment achieve maximum independence and quality of life. It encompasses a range of services and strategies designed to address the unique needs and challenges associated with vision loss.

Occupational Therapy evaluation:

Participation in play, self-care, school occupations, and preparation for work are areas of focus for evaluation depending on the age and needs of the child.

Evaluation of the performance skills that support or limit the child's ability to engage in daily activities, and the activity demands, client factors, and contexts in which the child performs these activities, is a part of a comprehensive assessment.

Occupational Therapist work on the following:

- Develop Self-care skills
- Enhance Sensory Processing, Sensory Modulation and Sensory Integration
- Enhance Postural Control
- Develop body awareness & spatial orientation
- Develop tactile - proprioceptive perceptual abilities
- Maximize use of Functional vision
- Strengthen cognitive skills
- Enhance auditory perceptual skills

Occupational Therapy Visual Rehabilitation: Seven-Steps Sequential Treatment Plan

- Optimizing Client Factors
- Optimizing Context and teaching a client to modify the context
- Teaching Non- Visual Skills
    - Learn to use non-visual devices, techniques (Tactile, Auditory, Olfactory) and Cognition
    - Physical Movement and exploration without vision
    - Orientation
    - Sensory concept development and compensation
    - Optimize social context
    - Self- Regulation
    - Braille
- Teaching use of visual skills
    - Fixation, Localisation, Scanning and Tracking
    - Eccentric viewing
    - Visual Scanning
    - Visual Skill training without then with a device

- Education
    - Nature of eye disease
    - Outlook for the future
    - Expectations of vision rehabilitation
- Therapeutic Activities
    - Eccentric Viewing
    - Scanning
    - Reading skills
- Environmental Modifications
    - Lighting
    - Contrast
    - Glare
    - Size
    - Distance
    - Colour
- Non-optical Assistive Devices
    - Visual
    - Tactile
    - Auditory
- Optical Magnification
- Computer Technology in Low Vision Rehabilitation
- Resource/ Handouts

Summary

Occupational Therapist provide highly individualized/tailored made interventions to the specific needs, goals, and preferences of each person with visual impairment. Occupational Therapy helps individuals achieve greater independence and an improved quality of life by addressing their functional needs.

Chapter 18

RHEUMATOLOGY

Introduction

Rheumatology focuses on the diagnosis and treatment of conditions and diseases that affect the musculoskeletal system and autoimmune disorders.

Rheumatologists focus on a wide range of conditions, including various forms of arthritis, autoimmune diseases, and musculoskeletal pain disorders.

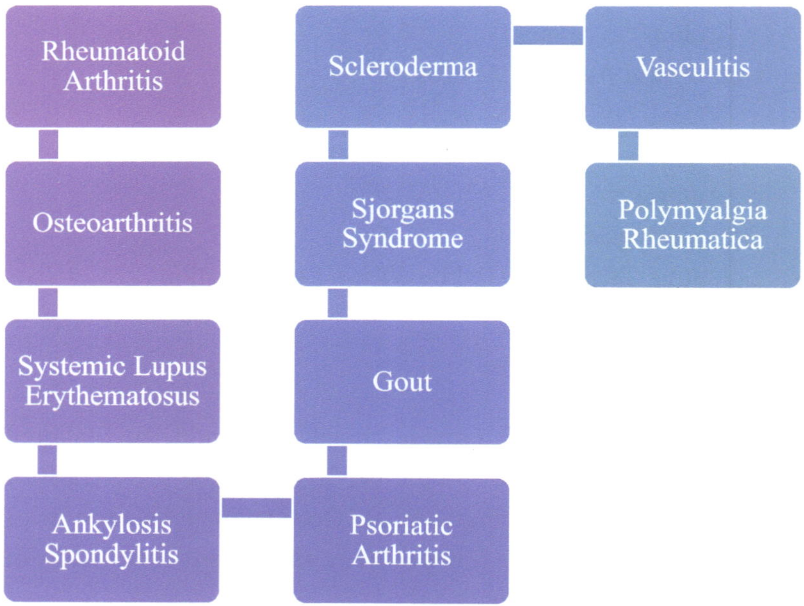

Occupational Therapy Role in Rheumatology

The role of Occupational Therapy in Rheumatology is holistic, aiming to improve an individual's overall well-being, enhance their quality of life, and enable them to participate in meaningful activities despite the challenges posed by rheumatic diseases.

- Assessment
- Pain Mangement
- Self-Management
- Functional Independence
- Activity Modification
- Energy conservation
- Joint Protection
- Emotional Support
- Assisstive devices
- Home & Work Environment Modification

- **Assessment:** The Occupational Therapy assessment includes evaluating physical, emotional, and functional aspects.
- **Education:** Occupational Therapists educate patients about their condition, its management, and the importance of self-care.
- **Joint Protection:** Occupational Therapists teach patients techniques to protect their joints from further damage.
- **Activity Modification:** Occupational Therapists work with individuals to modify or adapt daily activities and routines by recommending changes in how tasks are performed to make them more manageable and less painful.

- **Pain Management:** Modalities like heat and cold therapy, splinting, and providing guidance on relaxation and breathing techniques are suggested by Occupational Therapist.
- **Functional Independence:** Occupational Therapists work on improving mobility, dexterity, and strength to enable individuals to perform essential activities such as dressing, grooming, cooking, and bathing which will enhance their functional independence.
- **Assistive Devices:** Occupational Therapists recommend assistive devices such as adaptive utensils, reachers, dressing aids, and mobility aids like canes or walkers and many more.
- **Home and Work Environment Modification:** Occupational Therapists assess home and work environments to identify hazards and suggest modifications to provide safer and more accessible environment.
- **Energy Conservation:** Occupational Therapists teach energy conservation strategies to help individuals manage their energy levels and prioritize important activities.
- **Emotional Support:** Occupational Therapists provide emotional support and coping strategies to address the psychological aspects of the condition.
- **Self-Management:** Occupational Therapists empower individuals to take an active role in managing their condition. They help patients by setting goals, develop action plans, and monitor their progress.

Summary

Occupational Therapy plays a vital role in the field of Rheumatology by helping individuals with rheumatic conditions effectively manage their symptoms, improve their quality of life, and maintain their independence in daily activities.

Chapter 19

DERMATOLOGY

Introduction

Dermatology is a medical specialty that focuses on the diagnosis, treatment, and management of conditions and diseases related to the skin, hair, nails, and mucous membranes.

Occupational Therapy play a valuable role in dermatology by helping individuals with skin conditions and dermatological concerns improve their daily functioning, manage symptoms, and enhance their overall quality of life. While dermatology primarily focuses on diagnosing and treating skin disorders, Occupational Therapy complements these efforts by addressing the functional and psychosocial aspects of living with a skin condition.

Skin Condition that affects Psychosocial well-being

- Vitiligo
- Acne
- Psoriasis
- Eczema
- Herpes Simplex
- Skin cancer
- Fungal infections

Here are some ways in which Occupational Therapy can be beneficial in dermatology

- **Skin Care Education:** Occupational Therapists educate individuals on proper skincare routines, wound care, and techniques for managing specific skin conditions. They provide guidance on selecting appropriate skin care products, preventing skin irritations, and maintaining skin hygiene.

- **Psychosocial Support:** Skin conditions can have a significant impact on an individual's self-esteem, body image, and emotional well-being. Occupational Therapists offer emotional support and coping strategies to help individuals manage the psychological aspects of living with a skin condition.
- **Pain Management:** Some dermatological conditions, such as chronic skin disorders or wounds, can be painful. Occupational Therapists teach pain management techniques, including relaxation techniques and positioning strategies, to help individuals alleviate discomfort and improve their ability to perform daily activities.
- **Scar Management:** After surgical procedures or injuries that result in scarring, Occupational Therapists provide scar management techniques and strategies to improve scar mobility, appearance, and function.
- **Assistive Devices and Adaptive Strategies:** Occupational Therapists assess an individual's needs for assistive devices or adaptive equipment to aid in Activities of Daily Living (ADLs) and ensure independence despite physical limitations caused by skin conditions.
- **Occupational Analysis:** Occupational Therapists perform assessments to understand how a skin condition impacts a person's ability to engage in meaningful occupations and activities. Then they develop personalized intervention plans to address these limitations.
- **Occupational Rehabilitation:** For individuals with work-related skin conditions, Occupational Therapists collaborate with employers to modify work environments, provide ergonomic recommendations, and design return-to-work programs to support employees in their Occupational roles.

- **Patient Education:** Occupational Therapists educate patients about lifestyle modifications, such as dietary changes, stress management techniques, and sun protection measures, that help manage and prevent skin conditions.
- **Wound Care Management:** Occupational Therapists assist individuals with chronic wounds or dermatological conditions that require wound care by teaching them how to clean, dress, and protect wounds properly.
- **Adherence to Treatment Plans:** Occupational Therapists work with individuals to enhance adherence to dermatological treatment plans, ensuring that prescribed medications, topical treatments, and lifestyle changes are followed consistently.

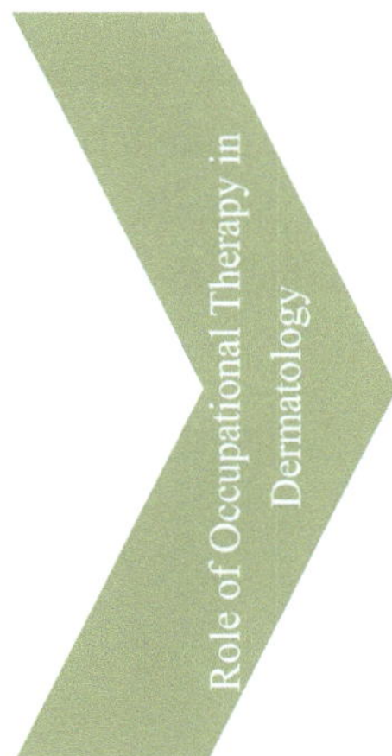

- Patient Education
- Skin Care Education
- Psychosocial Support
- Wound Care Management
- Scar management
- Pain Management
- Assistive & Adaptive devices
- Occupational Analysis
- Occupational Rehabilitation

Summary

Occupational Therapist play a very important role in Dermatology and its related conditions by focusing on their daily functioning, psychosocial well-being and overall Quality of Life.

Chapter 20

ONCOLOGY AND PALLIATIVE CARE

Introduction

Cancer is a complex group of diseases characterized by the uncontrolled growth and spread of abnormal cells in the body. These abnormal cells, known as cancer cells, can form masses or tumours that invade nearby tissues and organs. If left untreated or uncontrolled, cancer can eventually lead to serious health problems and, in some cases, become life-threatening.

Cancer is a significant public health concern worldwide, and ongoing research continues to improve our understanding of its causes, prevention, and treatment. Early detection, lifestyle choices, and advances in medical science have contributed to improved survival rates for many types of cancer

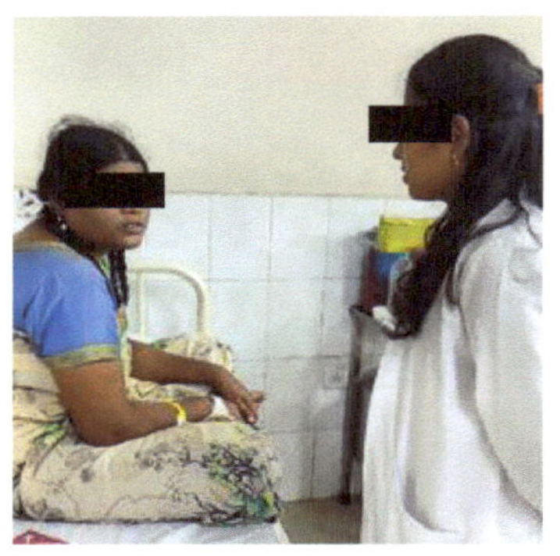

(a) Functional Status Screening

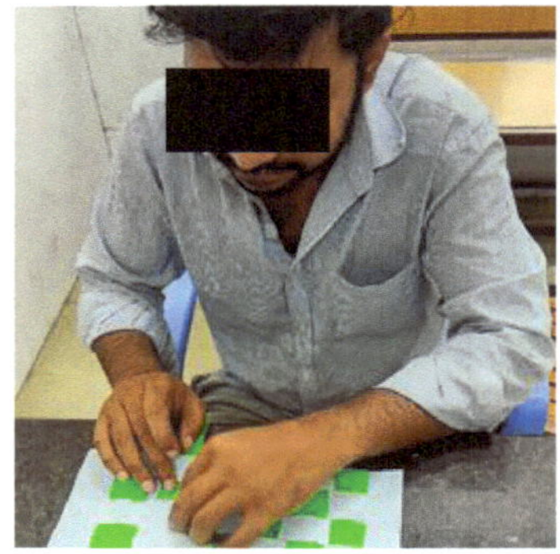

(b) Recreational Activity

Role of Occupational Therapy in Oncology

Occupational Therapists aim to improve Quality of Life, so that peoples' lives will be as comfortable and productive and live independent as possible. This applies even if life expectancy is short. Because people with cancer can experience very rapid changes in their illness and care setting.

Occupational Therapists working with patients with cancer be particularly responsive to changing needs. They respond quickly and plan forward carefully to take account of deterioration. Occupational Therapists have a role to play at all stages of the cancer, from diagnosis to Palliative and Terminal care.

Occupational Therapists promote the well-being and independence of people with cancer in various settings:

- Home Environment
- Hospital Setting (acute or community)
- Nursing and Residential homes
- Daycare Hospices
- In-patient hospices

Screening and Assessment

Occupational Therapists will work through the following sequence:

- Initial Interview
- Occupational Therapy Assessment
- Identifying abilities and needs of the Patient
- Goal setting (short term & long term)
- Providing Intervention
- Ongoing assessment
- Revision of Intervention plan
- Measurement of Therapy Outcome
- Follow-up
- Home program

Caregiver well-being

Caregiver well-being has both direct and indirect effects on the quality of cancer care, including support received from the health care team, the caregiver themselves, and in relation to the patient's daily activities.

Occupational Therapy Intervention

- ADL Management
- Occupational Engagement/Vocational Resettlement
- Psychosocial Support
- Environmental Modification
- Providing Assistive and Adaptive Devices
- Contracture Management after surgery
- Relaxation Techniques
- Scar Management
- Energy Conservation Techniques
- Pain Management
- Fatigue Management
- Group Therapy
- Lifestyle Modification
- Work Simplification Techniques

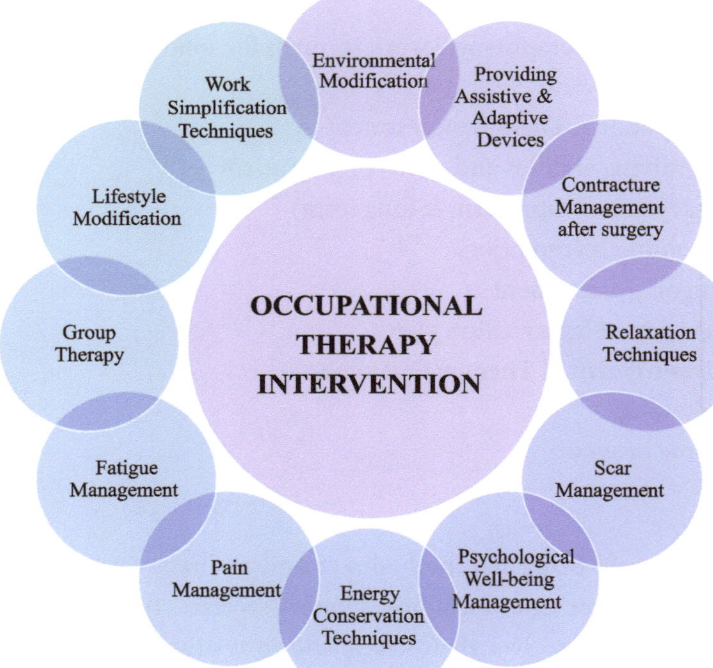

Occupational Therapy Intervention Approaches in Oncology

Cancer Rehabilitation Paradigms	Focus of Paradigm Intervention	Occupational Therapy Intervention Approaches	Focus of Occupational Therapy Interventions
Preventive	• Pre-operative training • Improve general health and function.	• Prevent (disability prevention)	• To prevent the occurrence or evolution of barriers to performance in context.
Restorative	• Return to previous levels of function.	• Establish, restore (remediation, restoration) • Prevent	• To change client variables to establish a skill or ability that has not yet developed or to restore a skill or ability that has been impaired.
Supportive	• Accommoda-tion training for existing disabilities. • Minimize potential debilitating changes.	• Modify (compensation, adaptation) • Prevent • Maintain	• To find ways to revise the current context or activity demands to support performance in the natural setting.
Palliative	• Best quality of life for client and family. • Balance between function and comfort.	• Maintain • Modify	• To provide the supports that will allow the client to preserve the performance capabilities that have been regained, to continue to meet the client's occupational needs, or both. • Assumption: without continued maintenance intervention, performance would decrease, occupational needs would not be met, or both, thereby affecting health and quality of life.

Cancer Rehabilitation Paradigms: Occupational Therapy Role

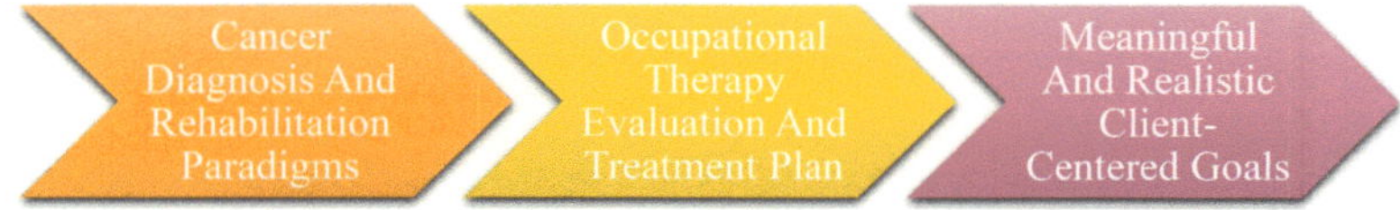

Summary

Occupational Therapy Intervention in Cancer rehabilitation focuses on functional independence of the patients. Occupational Therapist promotes Psychological well-being aiming to improve a better Quality Of Life to the patients.

Chapter 21

GERIATRICS

Role of Occupational Therapy in Geriatrics

Occupational Therapists help seniors lead active and independent lives. Occupational Therapists help them to perform daily activities independently using compensatory strategies.

Geriatric Conditions Relevant to Occupational Therapy

- Cardiovascular Problems
- Cerebrovascular Accidents (CVA)
- Cancer and Related Problems
- Diabetes Mellitus
- Arthritis
- Age-related Visual and Hearing Impairments
- Dementia and Alzheimer's Disease
- Parkinson's Disease
- Late - life Psychosis
- Mood and Anxiety Disorders
- Urinary Incontinence
- Psychological impact of aging

Occupational Therapy Settings

- Gerio-Psychiatric Unit
- Inpatient / Outpatient Rehabilitation
- Adult Foster Home
- Assisted Living Facility Centre
- Home Health Agency
- Hospice Facility Centre
- Adult Day Care
- Community Wellness Care

Role of Occupational Therapy

- **Screening and Evaluation:** Occupational Therapists conduct comprehensive assessments to identify an older individual's physical, cognitive, sensory, and psychosocial abilities and limitations. This evaluation helps in understanding their specific needs and developing a personalized treatment plan.
- **Activities of Daily Living (ADL):** Occupational Therapists work with older adults to maintain or regain independence in basic self-care activities, including bathing, dressing, grooming, toileting, and feeding.
- **Instrumental Activities of Daily Living (IADLs):** These are more complex tasks related to independent living, such as meal preparation, housekeeping, medication management, and managing finances. Occupational Therapists help seniors improve their ability to perform these activities.
- **Fall Prevention:** Falls are a significant concern for the elderly. They also provide activities and strategies to improve balance and mobility.
- **Home Safety and Modifications:** Occupational Therapists assess the home environment and suggest modifications or adaptations to make the living space more accessible and safer for older adults.
- **Cognitive Rehabilitation:** For seniors with cognitive impairments, Occupational Therapists provide cognitive retraining to address memory, attention, problem-solving, and executive function deficits.
- **Upper Extremity Rehabilitation:** Occupational Therapists design programs to improve the strength and coordination of the hands and arms, allowing seniors to maintain or regain skills required for activities like dressing, eating, and grooming.
- **Assistive Devices and Technology:** Occupational Therapists recommend and train older adults in the use of adaptive equipment and assistive devices, such as mobility aids, hearing aids, and communication devices, to enhance independence.

- **Community Engagement and Social Participation:** Occupational Therapists work with seniors to maintain or establish social connections, participate in community activities, and pursue hobbies and interests that contribute to a sense of purpose and well-being.
- **Psychosocial Support:** Aging can bring emotional and psychological challenges. Occupational Therapists provide emotional support and strategies for coping with issues like depression, anxiety, and isolation.
- **Caregiver Education and Support:** Occupational Therapists often work with family members and caregivers, providing them with education and training on how to best support and assist older adults with their unique needs.
- **Transition Planning:** In cases where a senior is transitioning from a hospital or rehabilitation facility back to their home, Occupational Therapists assist with the planning and adaptation of the living environment.

Interventions for Geriatric

- Activities to promote Physical and Mental health Well-being
- Fall prevention programs
- Addressing memory problems
- ADL Scheduling and training
- Recreational activities
- Providing Assistive and adaptive devices
- Environment/home Assessment and modifications or adaptations
- Safety measures and precautions
- Energy conservation and Work simplification techniques
- Pain management Strategies.
- Recommendations for coping with hearing and visual impairments
- Adaptations for elderly with incontinence
- Hospice and palliative care
- Group therapy and Family therapy

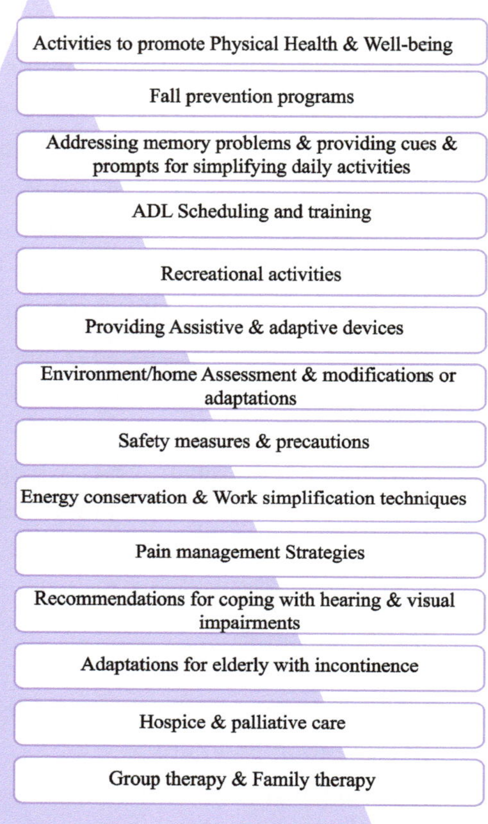

(Interventions For Geriatric Populations)

Summary

Occupational Therapists play a crucial role in enhancing the quality of life for the elderly, enabling them to live as independently as possible, and ensuring their safety and well-being. They work in various settings, including home care, rehabilitation centers, long-term care facilities, and outpatient clinics, collaborating with a multidisciplinary team of healthcare professionals to provide holistic care for older adults.

CHAPTER 22

REHABILITATION

Introduction

Occupational Therapy plays a critical role in rehabilitation, helping individuals regain independence and improve their quality of life after injury, illness, or disability. Here's a detailed explanation of the Occupational Therapy role in rehabilitation:

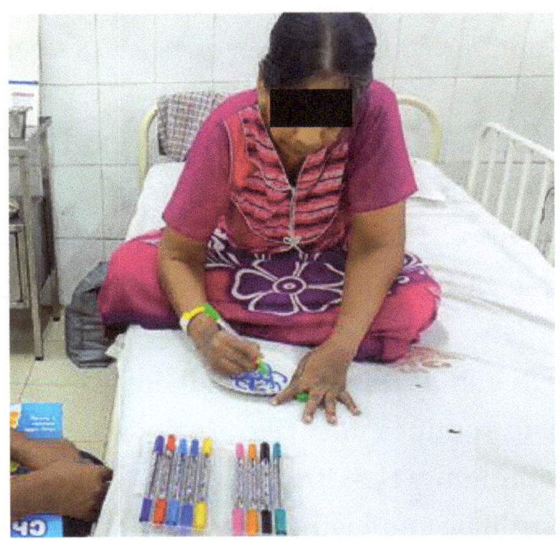

(a) Leisure Enhancement

Occupational Therapy role in rehabilitation

- **Comprehensive Assessment:** Occupational Therapists begin by conducting a thorough assessment of the individual. This assessment includes evaluating the person's physical, cognitive, emotional, and social capabilities, as well as their specific rehabilitation needs and goals.

- **Goal Setting:** Collaboratively set rehabilitation goals with the individual, taking into account their personal priorities and aspirations. Develop a customized treatment plan tailored to the person's goals, needs, and limitations.
- **Mobility and Motor Skills:** Focus on improving or restoring mobility, strength, balance, and coordination through targeted exercises and activities. Train individuals to use assistive devices like wheelchairs, walkers, or prosthetic limbs when necessary. Address issues related to posture and body mechanics.
- **Activities of Daily Living (ADLs):** Assist individuals in regaining independence in Activities of Daily Living (ADLs) such as bathing, dressing, grooming, and feeding. Teach adaptive techniques and provide assistive devices to enhance self-care skills.
- **Cognitive Rehabilitation:** Work with individuals who have cognitive impairments (e.g., brain injury or stroke) to improve memory, attention, problem-solving, and executive function. Provide strategies for managing cognitive challenges and promoting safety.
- **Functional Rehabilitation:** Help individuals regain or adapt to their roles and routines in society, including returning to work, school, or community activities. Provide vocational rehabilitation services to facilitate employment and job retention.
- **Assistive Technology:** Assess the need for and provide training in the use of assistive technology, such as communication devices or computer aids. Recommend home modification to enhance accessibility and safety.
- **Pain Management:** Develop strategies to manage pain through modalities, positioning, and activity modification. Educate individuals on pacing and energy conservation techniques to prevent exacerbation of pain.
- **Emotional Support and Coping:** Offer emotional support and coping strategies to address psychological challenges associated

with disability or illness. Facilitate support groups or mental health services when needed.

- **Home and Community Reintegration:** Assess the individual's ability to function safely at home and in the community. Provide training in community mobility and navigation skills to ensure a successful transition back to everyday life.
- **Family and Caregiver Education:** Educate family members and caregivers on how to support and assist the individual in their rehabilitation journey. Encourage collaboration and communication among the rehabilitation team and the individual's support network.
- **Follow-Up and Reassessment:** Conduct ongoing reassessments to track progress and adjust the treatment plan as needed. Ensure continuity of care and provide long-term support as required.

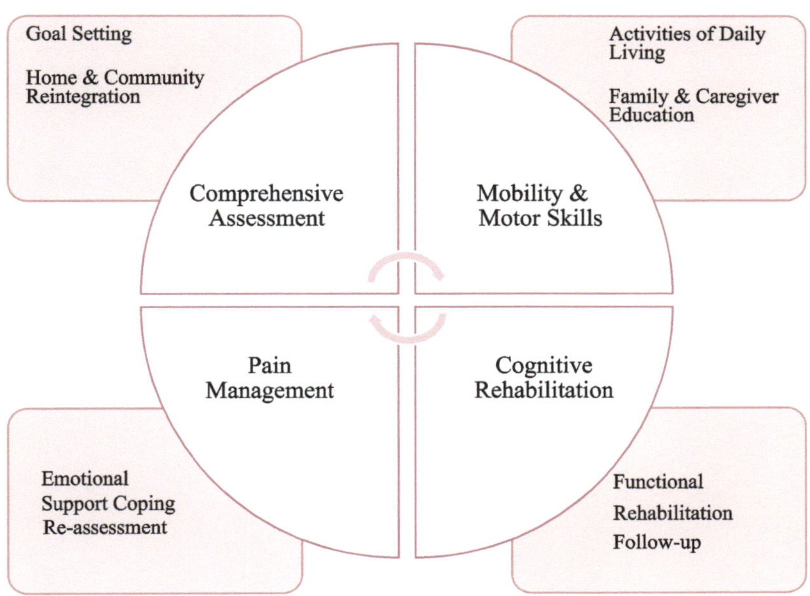

Summary

Occupational Therapy in rehabilitation is a client-centred and holistic approach that addresses physical, cognitive, emotional, and social aspects of recovery. Occupational Therapy aim to promote functional independence, enhance quality of life, and empower individuals to participate fully in their chosen roles and activities, regardless of their physical or cognitive challenges. Rehabilitation is often a collaborative effort among various healthcare professionals, with Occupational Therapists playing a central role in optimizing outcomes and maximizing independence for individuals on their path to recovery.

CHAPTER 23

COMMUNITY BASED REHABILITATION (CBR)

Introduction

Community-Based Occupational Therapy practice revolves around the social participation (social roles and meaningful activities) of the individual, group, or community. It focuses on the client's health promotion and prevention, community participation, and empowerment.

Occupational Therapy and Community-Based Rehabilitation (CBR) share many similarities in their objectives and methods. Both emphasize the value of increasing the welfare and engagement of people with disabilities in their communities. One of the fields that can be quite important in CBR programs is occupational therapy.

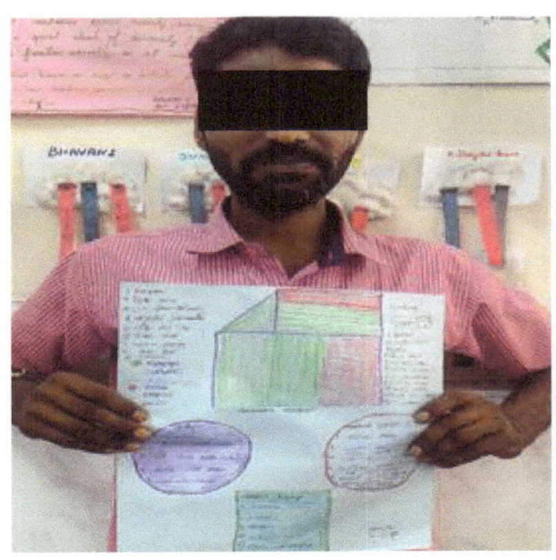

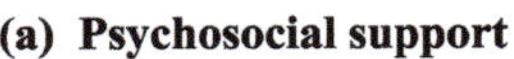

(a) Psychosocial support

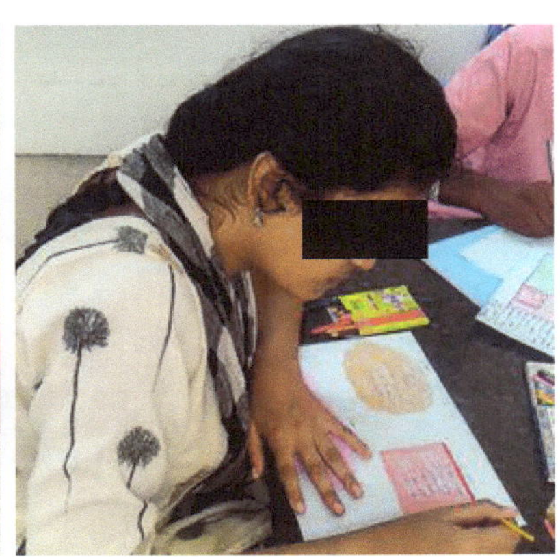

(b) Education and training

Role of Occupational Therapy

- Assessing individuals regarding Occupational engagement and participation
- Providing Client Education
- Addressing the client's unmet Health needs
- Serving the less privileged clients through health-related programs
- Promoting community inclusion
- Political advocacy
- Referral services

Occupational Therapy approach

- **Create and enhance health:** Provide contextual experiences and rich activities to improve people's performance in natural life contexts.
- **Establish, and restore health:** To change client variables to develop a skill or ability that has not yet been developed or to restore a skill or ability that has been impaired.
- **Maintain health:** To provide the support that will allow the client to maintain his/ her performance capabilities, thereby improving health and quality of life.
- **Modify, and adapt for health:** To find ways to revise the current context or activity demands to support performance through compensatory techniques, providing cues, or reducing distractibility.
- **Disability Prevention:** To prevent the occurrence of performance barriers in clients with or without a disability who are at risk for developing occupational performance problems.

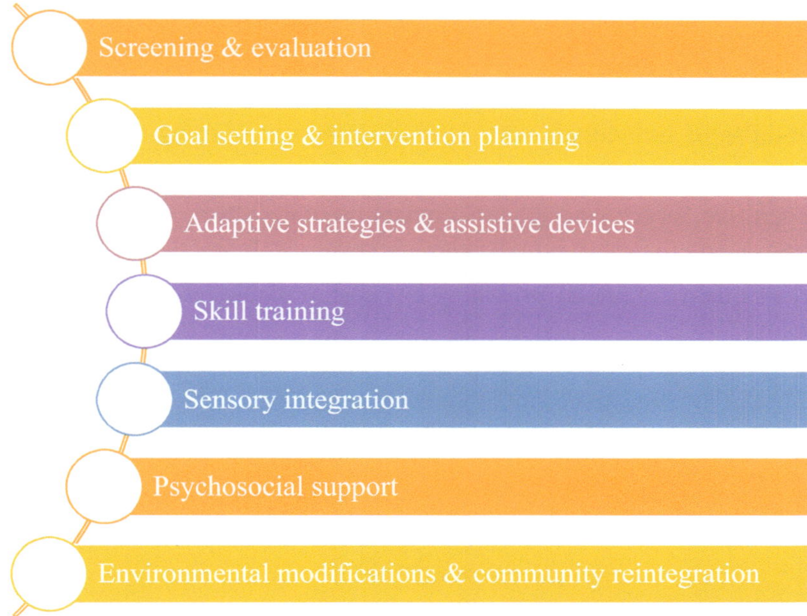

(Occupational Therapy in CBR)

Occupational Therapy interventions

- Health Literacy/ Client education on Physical and mental illness
- Leisure exploration and participation
- Stress management
- Relaxation techniques
- Sensory modulation
- Self- and peer-advocacy
- Community integration (engaging in the community as a contributing member)
- Pain management
- Physical Agent Modalities
- Ergonomics
- Home modification
- Recommending assistive and adaptive devices

Summary

Occupational Therapy is an integral component of community-based rehabilitation programs. It focuses on enhancing the functional abilities of individuals with disabilities and promoting their active participation within their communities. By addressing physical, cognitive, psychosocial, and environmental factors, Occupational Therapists help individuals achieve greater independence, improve their quality of life, by providing low cost avaliable resources.

Chapter 24

ACTIVITIES OF DAILY LIVING (ADL)

Introduction

Activities of Daily Living (ADL) are the tasks of self-maintenance, mobility, communication, and home management that enable an individual to achieve personal independence in his or her environment.

Occupational Therapy focuses on self-care activities and the improvement of fine motor coordination of muscles and joints, particularly in the upper extremities. Occupational Therapy focuses on Activities of Daily Living because they are the cornerstone of independent living.

BADL categories

BADL
Eating
Grooming
Bathing
Dressing
Toileting
Transfers
Locomotion
Sleep
Rest
Sexual Activity

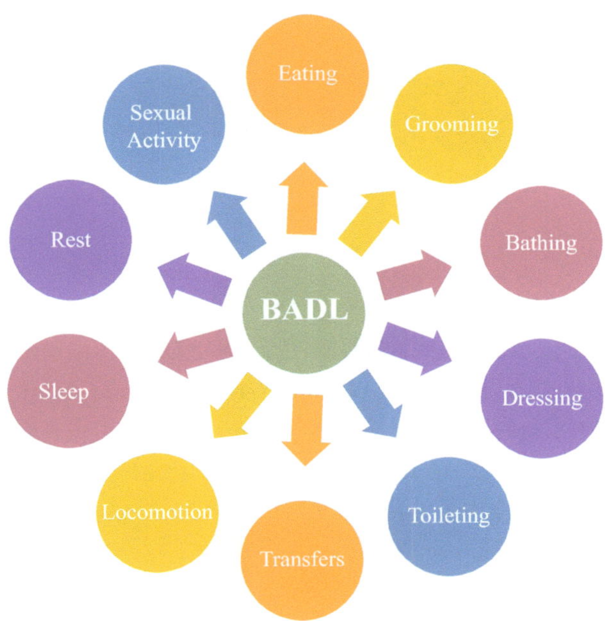

IADL categories

It requires more complex cognitive functioning than BADLs. It includes;

IADL
Ability to use Telephone
Shopping
Food Preparation
House keeping
Laundry
Mode of transportation
Responsibility for own Medications
Ability to handle finances
Safety & emergency maintenance
Religious Observance

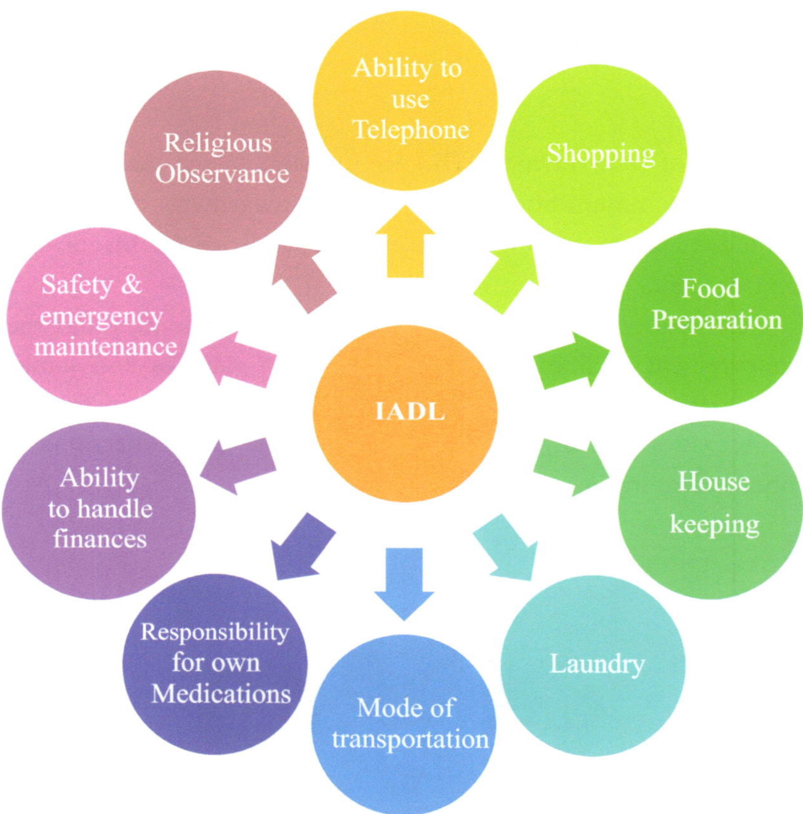

Causes for limitations in ADLs

Limitations in Activities of Daily Living (ADLs) can result from a variety of factors, including physical, cognitive, and environmental issues. ADLs are essential tasks necessary for independent living, and limitations in these activities can significantly impact a person's ability to care for themselves. Here are some common causes of limitations in ADLs:

Causes of Limitations to ADLs

Physical Disabilies

Cognitive Impairment

Mental Health Issues

Aging

Neurological conditions

Environmental Factors

Evaluation

Patients are evaluated for limitations that require intervention and for strengths that can be used to compensate for weaknesses. Limitations may involve motor function, sensation, cognition, or psychosocial function. Examiners determine which activities (e.g., work, leisure, social, learning) patients want or need help with. Patients need help with a general type of activity (e.g., social) or a specific activity (e.g., attending church), or they need to be motivated to do an activity.

Therapists use an assessment instrument to help in the evaluation. Occupational Therapists assess the home for hazards and make recommendations to ensure home safety (e.g., removing throw rugs, increasing hallway and kitchen lighting, moving a night table within reach of the bed, and placing a family picture on a door to help patients recognize their room).

Occupational Therapy in ADL training

- Skill Training
- Visual Demonstration
- Assistive technology
- Adaptive Devices
- Home & Environmental modification

Summary

Occupational Therapy is a client-centered profession that aims to improve an individual's overall quality of life by enabling them to participate in the activities that are important to them. The specific interventions and goals of Occupational Therapy will vary depending on the client's needs, goals, and the challenges they face in their daily life.

Chapter 25

SPORTS

Introduction

Sports are a fundamental aspect of human culture and society that cut across all demographics, including all ages and socioeconomic levels. They cover a wide range of physical pursuits and sports that demand effort, skill, and competition. Sports have a huge impact on uniting people, fostering physical fitness, and advancing values like teamwork, discipline, and sportsmanship from ancient civilizations to the present.

Beyond the recreational and entertainment aspects, sports can instill essential life skills and values. Participation in sports teaches individuals teamwork, leadership, perseverance, and the importance of fair play. It provides opportunities for personal growth, physical fitness, and the pursuit of excellence.

What Do Occupational Therapists Do?

Occupational Therapy contribute significantly to sports and athletics, despite the fact that it is less frequently connected to sports than other healthcare specialties like physical Therapy or sports medicine. But Occupational Therapists make a variety of positive contributions to athletes' health and performance. Occupational Therapy employs a holistic approach to include the client's roles and environment in addition to the factors that have influenced their ability to participate in activities.

The approach focuses on three areas:

- Wellness promotion
- Rehabilitation
- Habilitation

Types

Sports injuries are broadly categorized into two kinds:

- Acute injuries, which happen suddenly.
- Chronic injuries, which are usually related to overuse and develop gradually over time.

Common Sports Injuries

- Bone fracture
- Dislocation
- Sprain
- Strain
- Tendinitis
- Bursitis
- Knee injuries
- Rotator cuff injuries
- Tennis elbow
- Golfer's elbow
- ACL tear
- Sciatica

Injuries can occur suddenly, without warning or gradually over time due to overuse. Each sport has different risks of injury on its players.

Intervention Strategies

Injury Prevention and Management

- Occupational Therapist assess an athlete's biomechanics, ergonomics, and equipment use to identify potential risk factors for injuries. They provide recommendations for injury prevention strategies.
- In the event of an injury, Occupational Therapist assist with rehabilitation by developing customized exercise and mobility programs to help athletes regain their functional abilities.

Performance Enhancement

- Occupational Therapists work with athletes to optimize their physical and cognitive performance. This includes improving strength, endurance, flexibility, and coordination to enhance athletic skills.
- They also help athletes develop strategies for managing stress, anxiety, and performance-related mental health issues.

Return to Sport

- After a sports-related injury, Occupational Therapists assist athletes in their return-to-sport process. This involves evaluating functional abilities and working on a gradual return to physical activity to ensure safety and minimize the risk of re-injury.

Pain Management

- Occupational Therapists provide pain management strategies and techniques, including modalities like heat and cold therapy, splinting, to help athletes manage pain and discomfort related to sports injuries or conditions.

Adaptive Sports

- Occupational Therapists often play a crucial role in adaptive sports programs, working with individuals who have physical or cognitive disabilities to engage in sports and recreational activities adapted to their abilities.
- They work with athletes to customize equipment, such as adaptive wheelchairs or prosthetic devices, to meet their specific needs.

Wellness and Lifestyle Coaching

- Occupational Therapists offer guidance on maintaining a healthy lifestyle, including nutrition, sleep, stress management, and overall well-being, which can benefit athletes in their training and performance.

Injury Prevention & Management
Performance Enhancement
Return to Sport
Pain Management
Adaptive Sports
Wellness & Lifestyle Coaching

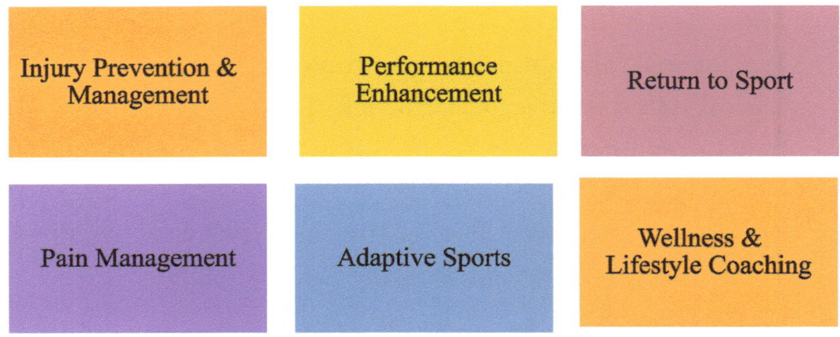

(Role of Occupational Therapy in Sports)

Summary

Overall, Occupational Therapists contribute to the holistic care of athletes by addressing their physical, mental, and functional needs. Their role in sports may vary depending on the athlete's specific goals, needs, and the nature of the sport. Collaborative efforts with other healthcare professionals, such as physical therapists, sports medicine physicians, and coaches, are often essential to provide comprehensive care for athletes.

Chapter 26

LEISURE

Introduction

Occupational Therapy is essential for aiding people of all ages in engaging in meaningful leisure activities. A person's existence is not complete without leisure because it promotes their physical, emotional, and social well-being. Here are some ways that leisure and Occupational Therapy interact.

The absence of productive leisure can have negative consequences on a person's physical and mental health, as well as their personal development, social relationships, and general well-being. Leading a balanced and fulfilled life may include supporting and making time for worthwhile leisure pursuits.

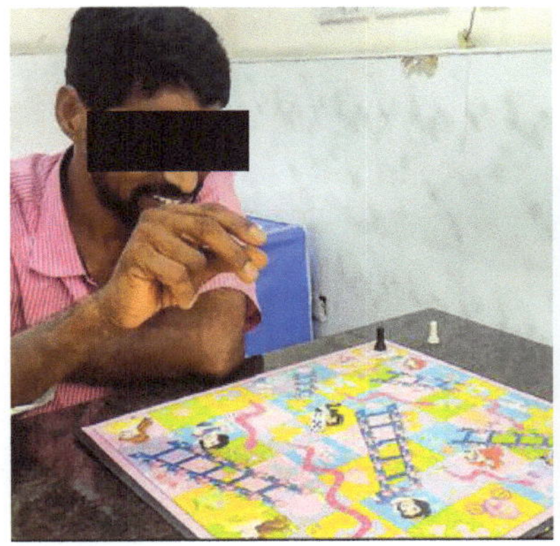

(a) Problem Solving Games

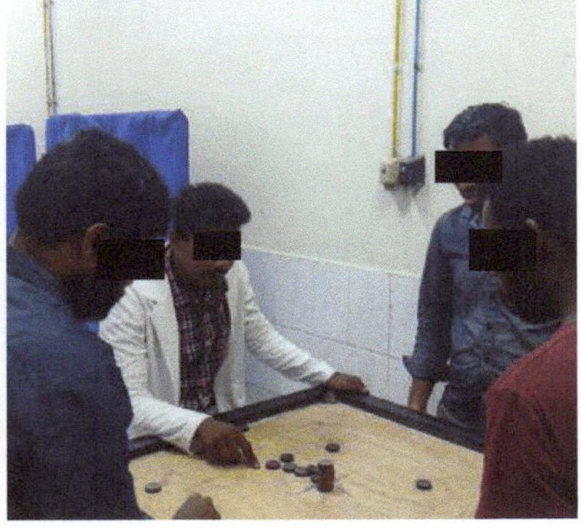

(b) Goal Enhancement

Assessment and Evaluation

- Occupational Therapists assess an individual's physical, cognitive, emotional, and social capabilities to determine their interests, strengths, and limitations related to leisure activities.

- They use standardized assessments to identify areas where a person may benefit from therapeutic interventions to enhance leisure participation.

Goal Setting

- Occupational Therapists work with clients to set specific, client-centered goals related to leisure participation.
- These goals range from improving fine motor skills for a hobby like painting to enhancing cognitive abilities for card games or adapting equipment for sports and recreation

Skill Development

- Occupational Therapists provide interventions to help individuals develop or regain the necessary skills and abilities required for leisure activities.
- This involves physical rehabilitation, cognitive training, sensory integration, or social skills development, depending on the individual's needs.

Adaptation and Modification

- Occupational Therapist often adapt or modify leisure activities and equipment to make them accessible to individuals with disabilities or limitations.
- They recommend adaptive tools, assistive devices, or environmental modifications to ensure safe and enjoyable participation in leisure pursuits.

Time Management and Routine Building

- Occupational Therapists help clients manage their time effectively to include leisure activities within their daily routines.
- They work on establishing balanced routines that prioritize self-care, work, and leisure to promote overall well-being.

Stress Reduction and Coping

- Leisure activities serve as a valuable means of stress reduction and emotional regulation.
- Occupational Therapists teach relaxation techniques and coping strategies through leisure activities such as yoga, meditation, or mindfulness practices.

Social Engagement

- Leisure activities often involve social interaction and community engagement.
- Occupational Therapists work on improving social skills, communication, and interpersonal relationships to enhance a person's ability to participate in group leisure activities.

Quality of Life Enhancement

- In the end, Occupational Therapy aims to enhance a person's quality of life by enabling them to take part in satisfying and pleasurable leisure activities.
- This lead to better psychological well-being, self-worth, and overall satisfaction.

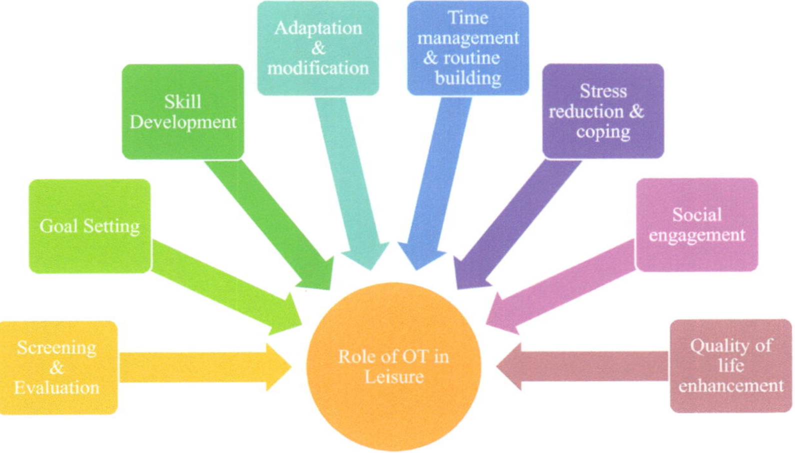

(Role of Occupational Therapy in Leisure)

Summary

By appreciating the importance of leisure activities in a person's life, Occupational Therapists make substantial contributions to the promotion of a holistic approach to health and wellbeing. They encourage individuals in overcoming barriers, adjusting to constraints, and fully engaging in leisure activities that enrich, fulfil, and give meaning to their lives.

Chapter 27

VOCATIONAL REHABILITATION

Introduction

Vocational rehabilitation essentially involves preparing for work, applying for jobs, and getting a job. The goal of vocational rehabilitation is to help people achieve functional, psychological, developmental, cognitive, and emotional disabilities or overcome access barriers for people with disabilities. Maintain or return to work or any other useful occupation.

Our leadership role

The goal of Occupational Therapy therefore clearly includes vocational rehabilitation that addresses one of these three life domains, including practical and goal-directed interventions that promote recovery and overcome barriers to work participation.

We offer the following services

- Assess and treat the individual to maximize their work ability.
- Assess the home and work environment and make recommendations regarding equipment or adaptations to support the individual to continue working.
- Provide the person with information and links to other important resources that can support them. For example: other professionals, other agencies, hardware resources, information about their health status, or information about legislation that supports them.
- Lifestyle management skills, i.e., Create daily routines, use public transport, etc.
- Create trust.

- Participation in a group program.
- Symptom management / mental health monitoring.

Occupational Therapy in vocational rehabilitation is a collaborative process that involves working closely with vocational counsellors, employers, and other healthcare professionals to create customized plans that maximize an individual's potential for successful employment. It focuses on not just securing a job but also on ensuring long-term job retention and career advancement for people with disabilities or functional limitations.

How Occupational Therapy contributes to vocational rehabilitation

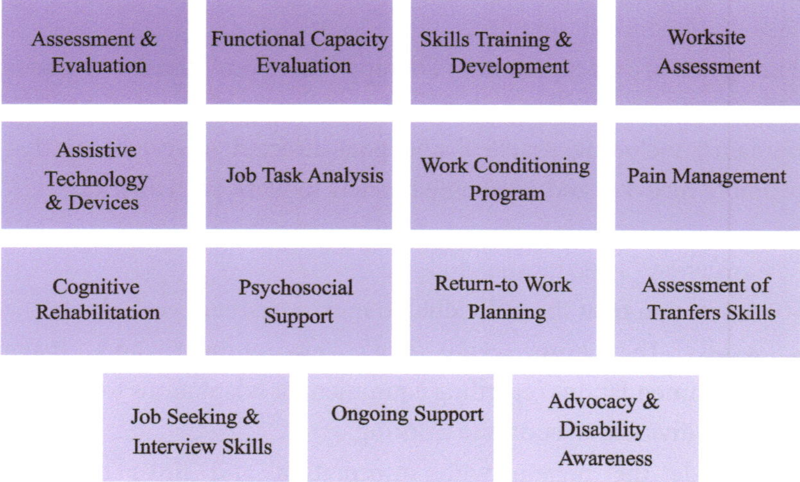

Summary

Occupational Therapy focuses on improving an individual's overall independence and functioning in daily life, while vocational rehabilitation specifically targets helping individuals with disabilities or barriers to employment enter or re-enter the workforce.

Chapter 28

ERGONOMICS

Introduction

Ergonomics (or human factors) is a discipline concerned with understanding the interaction between people and other parts of a system, and a profession that applies theory, principles, data and methods to design to optimize human comfort and well-being. When planning work and everyday situations, ergonomics focuses on the person. Unsafe, health-damaging, inconvenient or inefficient situations at work or in everyday life are avoided, considering the physical and psychological capabilities and limitations of a person.

Many factors affect ergonomics; these include body position and movement (sitting, standing, lifting, pulling and pushing), environmental factors (noise, vibration, lighting, climate, chemicals), information and performance (information received through vision or other senses, controls, touch screen and control), and work organization (correct tasks, interesting work). These factors greatly determine safety, health, comfort and efficient performance at work and in everyday life.

Ergonomics draws knowledge from various fields in the humanities and engineering sciences, including anthropometry, biomechanics, physiology, psychology, toxicology, mechanical engineering, industrial design, information technology, and management. It collected selected and integrated relevant information from these fields. Special methods and techniques are used to implement this knowledge.

Importance of Ergonomics

- **Health and well-being:** Ergonomics focuses primarily on optimizing the interaction between people and their environment. Proper ergonomic design can help reduce the risk of musculoskeletal disorders such as carpal tunnel syndrome, back pain and repetitive strain injuries. By promoting good posture and reducing physical stress, ergonomics improves physical health and overall well-being
- **Safety:** Ergonomics is closely related to safety in the workplace and other environments. When environments and tools are designed with ergonomics in mind, they are less likely to cause safety hazards. This way, accidents and incidents can be prevented, which makes workplaces and homes safer for everyone.
- **Productivity:** Ergonomically designed workspaces and tools can significantly increase productivity. When people feel comfortable and efficient at work, they work better and can maintain their ability to work longer. Reduced physical discomfort and fatigue also results in fewer rest breaks and less time due to health problems.
- **Comfort:** Ergonomics improves comfort in various environments, whether in the office, at home or in a vehicle. Comfortable seats, well-designed computer settings and ergonomic furniture add to a more pleasant and enjoyable experience.
- **Quality of life:** Ergonomics goes beyond the workplace. It influences the design of everyday objects, household appliances and even public spaces. Ergonomically designed products and environments improve the quality of life for people of all ages and abilities, making everyday tasks easier.
- **Accessibility and Inclusion:** Ergonomics plays an important role in making products and environments accessible to people with disabilities. It promotes inclusion and equal opportunities for people with different physical and cognitive abilities.

- **Cost savings:** Although there may be initial costs associated with ergonomic design, the long-term benefits often outweigh them. Fewer workplace accidents, lower healthcare costs, increased productivity and reduced absenteeism can result in significant savings for businesses and organizations.

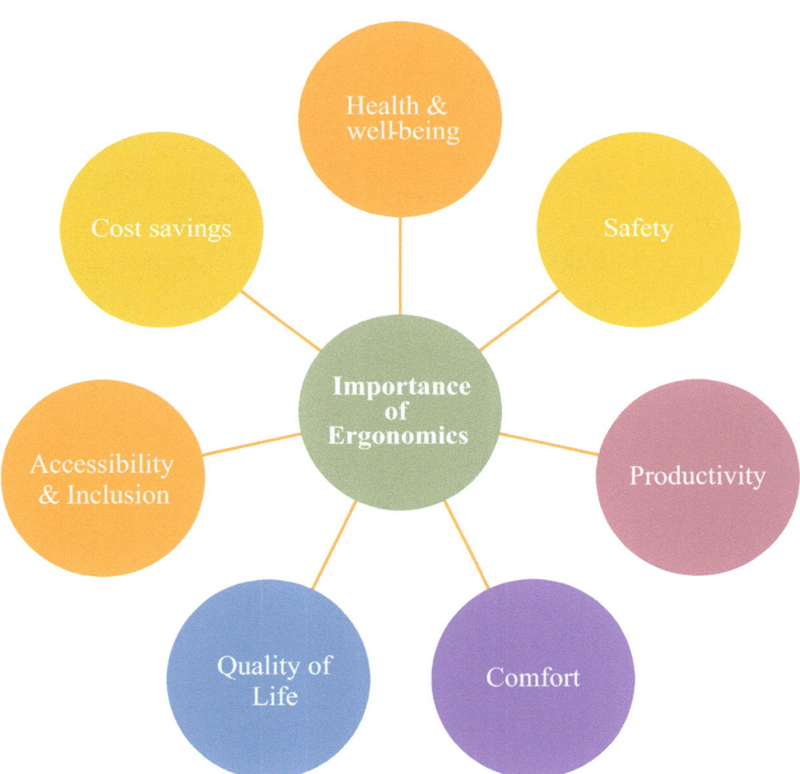

Occupational Therapy in Ergonomics

Occupational Therapy plays an important role in the field of ergonomics, especially in promoting and improving the well-being and functionality of people in various environments, including the workplace. Occupational Therapists are trained professionals who focus on helping people with physical, cognitive or psychosocial problems to achieve maximum independence and quality of life.

- Assessment and Evaluation
- Customized Ergonomic Solutions
- Education and Training
- Rehabilitation and Return-to-Work Programs
- Wellness Promotion

Summary

Ergonomics is essential to promote health, safety, productivity and overall quality of life. Ergonomic Occupational Therapy focuses on improving people's ability to perform tasks safely and effectively in their environment. By addressing ergonomic issues and tailoring interventions to individual needs, Occupational Therapists improve people's overall quality of life and ability to function in a variety of work environments.

CHAPTER 29

ROBOTICS IN OCCUPATIONAL THERAPY

The Robotics in Occupational Therapy holds significant potential for enhancing therapeutic interventions and improving the quality of life for individuals with various physical and cognitive challenges.

Here are some ways in which Occupational Therapy and robotics may intersect in the future:

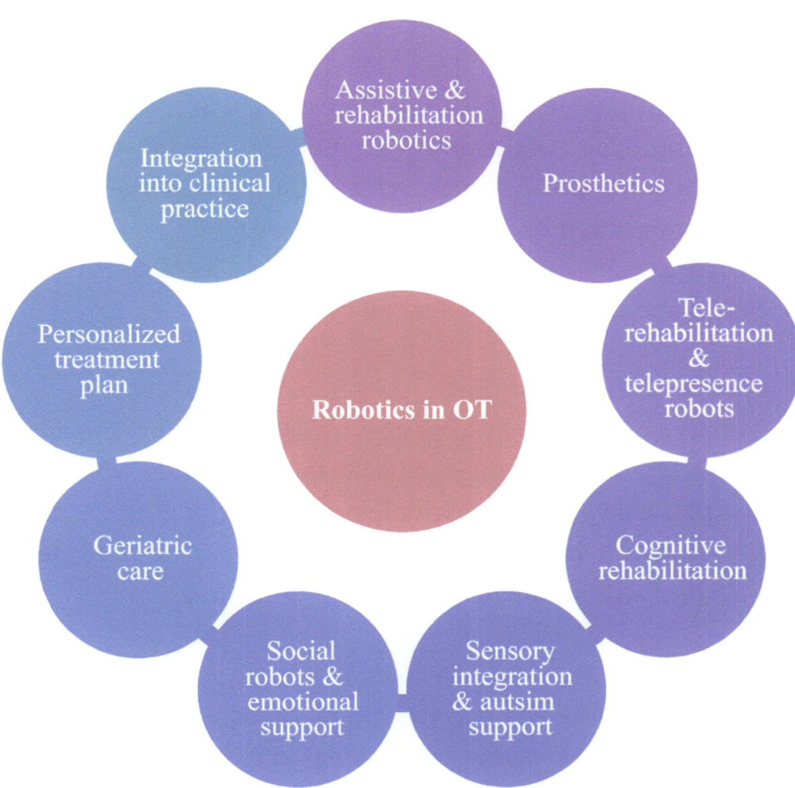

Assistive and Rehabilitation Robotics

- Advanced assistive robots help individuals who have difficulties to complete everyday tasks and exercises.
- Robots equipped with sensors and adaptive technologies provide real-time feedback and assistance during rehabilitation sessions.

Prosthetics and Exoskeletons

- Occupational Therapists work closely with individuals using advanced prosthetic limbs and exoskeletons.
- They help individuals adapt to and maximize the functionality of these devices, addressing the physical and psychosocial aspects of their use.

Tele-Rehabilitation and Telepresence Robots

- The utilization of telepresence robots by therapists to offer remote occupational therapy services through telerehabilitation programmes may become more widespread.
- People in remote places or those with limited mobility may have better access to therapy as a result of this.

Cognitive Rehabilitation

- Robots may assist in cognitive rehabilitation by providing interactive and engaging exercises for individuals with brain injuries, dementia, or cognitive impairments.
- Robots adapt tasks and challenges based on the individual's cognitive abilities and progress.

Sensory Integration and Autism Support

- Robots equipped with sensory integration capabilities may assist Occupational Therapists in working with individuals on the autism spectrum.

- These robots provide controlled sensory experiences to help individuals manage sensory sensitivities.

Social Robots for Emotional Support

- Social robots assist Occupational Therapists in addressing emotional and social challenges in Therapy.
- These robots engage individuals in social interactions, provide emotional support, and help build social skills.

Data and Analytics

- Robotics collect data on individuals' performance and progress during Therapy sessions.
- Occupational Therapists use this data to tailor interventions and measure outcomes more effectively.

Geriatric Care

- Occupational Therapists working with older adults may incorporate robotic technologies to support aging in place.
- Robots assist with activities such as medication management, fall detection, and communication with healthcare providers.

Personalized Treatment Plans

- Robotics, combined with artificial intelligence and machine learning, can help generate personalized treatment plans for individuals based on their specific needs and progress.

Integration into Clinical Practice

- Training programs for future Occupational Therapists may include education on how to effectively incorporate robotics into clinical practice.
- Occupational Therapists will need to adapt and learn how to utilize these technologies to enhance their therapeutic approaches.

Summary

While the integration of robotics into Occupational Therapy presents exciting possibilities, it's essential to strike a balance between technological advancements and the human touch and expertise that Occupational Therapists provide. Robotics in Occupational Therapy will likely involve ongoing research, collaboration with engineers and robotics experts, and a commitment to maintaining the client-centred and holistic principles that underpin the profession.

Chapter 30

VIRTUAL REALITY IN OCCUPATIONAL THERAPY

Virtual Reality in Occupational Therapy (VR) is an emerging and innovative approach that leverages VR technology to provide therapeutic interventions and support for individuals with various physical, cognitive, and emotional challenges.

Here are some key aspects of how Occupational Therapy is evolving with the integration of virtual-reality:

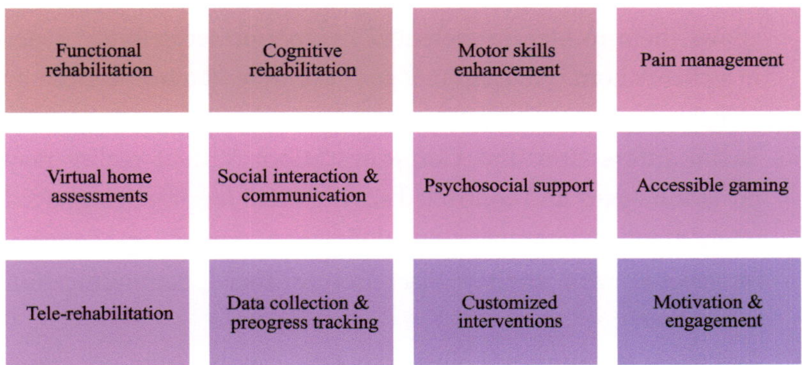

Virtual Reality in Occupational Therapy

- **Functional Rehabilitation:** Virtual reality can be used to create immersive environments that mimic real-life scenarios. Occupational Therapists design customized virtual reality experiences to help individuals practice and improve their daily living skills, such as cooking, dressing, or using public transportation.
- **Cognitive Rehabilitation:** Virtual reality environments can be tailored to address cognitive impairments, such as memory

deficits or attention difficulties. Therapists use VR-based cognitive training exercises to challenge and improve cognitive functions.

- **Motor Skills Enhancement:** Virtual reality systems equipped with motion-tracking sensors can aid in the development and refinement of fine and gross motor skills. Occupational Therapists use virtual reality to work on activities like hand-eye coordination, balance, and mobility.
- **Pain Management:** Virtual reality can serve as a distraction therapy tool for individuals experiencing pain or discomfort. By immersing patients in engaging virtual reality experiences, therapists help reduce the perception of pain and anxiety during therapy sessions.
- **Virtual Home Assessments:** Occupational Therapists conduct virtual home assessments using virtual reality technology. This allows them to identify potential hazards or accessibility issues in a client's home environment and recommend modifications or assistive devices.
- **Social Interaction and Communication:** Virtual reality may provide a secure and controlled environment for practicing social interactions, communication skills, and coping mechanisms for people with anxiety disorders or social communication difficulties.
- **Psychosocial Support:** Virtual reality can be used to create relaxation and mindfulness experiences to help individuals manage stress, anxiety, and emotional well-being. Therapists can guide clients through virtual reality -based meditation and relaxation exercises.
- **Accessible Gaming:** Accessible Virtual reality gaming platforms and experiences can be incorporated into therapy to motivate individuals and make rehabilitation more enjoyable. These games can be customized to address specific therapeutic goals.
- **Tele-Rehabilitation:** Virtual reality technology enables remote tele-rehabilitation services, allowing Occupational Therapists to

provide therapy sessions to clients who may not have access to in-person care.

- **Data Collection and Progress Tracking:** Virtual reality systems can collect data on an individual's performance within virtual environments. Therapists can use this data to track progress, tailor interventions, and make evidence-based decisions.
- **Customized Interventions:** Occupational Therapists have the flexibility to design and modify virtual reality experiences to suit each individual's unique needs and rehabilitation goals.
- **Motivation and Engagement:** The immersive and interactive nature of virtual reality can enhance motivation and engagement in therapy, especially for children and individuals with neurological conditions.

Summary

While Virtual reality holds great promise in Occupational Therapy, it's essential to ensure that Therapists are trained in the proper use of VR technology and that ethical considerations, safety, and individual preferences are taken into account. As the technology continues to advance, Occupational Therapy in virtual reality is likely to play an increasingly significant role in improving outcomes and enhancing the rehabilitation experience for clients of all ages and abilities.

Chapter 31

ARTIFICIAL INTELLIGENCE IN OCCUPATIONAL THERAPY

Introduction

Artificial Intelligence (AI) is characterized by the development of computer systems which has shown potential in healthcare and education for improving assessment and diagnostic processes, personalizing interventions, and enabling independent living.

Technology-based rehabilitation tools can be useful to organizations that have electronic data capture systems to monitor trends in rehabilitation service use and outcomes for quality improvement.

AI & OT

The integration of AI technologies in Occupational Therapy can enhance the delivery of individualized care, tailoring interventions to address specific needs. AI algorithms have been utilized to develop assessment tools capable of analysing data from various sources, supporting accurate evaluation of cognitive, physical, and emotional abilities

The AI based assessment tools empower Occupational Therapists to efficiently assess clients' needs and design personalized intervention plans. Additionally, Al- driven assistive technologies, such as robotic devices and smart home systems, have demonstrated promise in enhancing independence and quality of life for individuals with disabilities.

AI-driven assistive technologies

AI-driven assistive technologies have revolutionized the field of Occupational Therapy by leveraging artificial intelligence and machine learning algorithms to enhance independence, mobility, self-care, and environmental control for individuals with disabilities. These technologies offer innovative solutions that aim to improve the quality of life and promote inclusivity.

Personalized Interventions and Adaptive Learning

Personalized interventions and adaptive learning approaches have gained prominence in the field of Occupational Therapy. These approaches leverage AI technologies to tailor interventions according to individual needs, preferences, and progress. By incorporating personalized strategies and adaptive learning algorithms, these approaches aim to optimize therapeutic outcomes and enhance the effectiveness of interventions.

Summary

Artificial Intelligence (AI)-driven technologies have been developed to assist individuals in improving their communication skills, improving their functional independence, and engaging in meaningful social interactions enhancing their overall Quality of Life.

FREQUENTLY ASKED QUESTIONS IN OCCUPATIONAL THERAPY

- **Difference between Occupational Therapy and Physiotherapy?**

Aspect	Occupational Therapy (OT)	Physical therapy - (PT)
Primary Focus	Activities of Daily Living, Age Appropraite Skills, Psychosocial well-being through meaningful and purposeful actvities	Physical Funtion, Movement, Mobility through manual Therapy and Exercises

- **Does Occupational Therapy have PhD?**

Yes, some of the universities are offering Doctor of Philosophy (Ph. D) degree in Occupational Therapy. A Ph.D. in Occupational Therapy is typically pursued by individuals who are interested in advanced research, teaching, leadership roles, or academic careers within the field.

Ph.D. programs in Occupational Therapy are research-oriented and emphasize the development of advanced research skills. Students often conduct original research studies in areas related to Occupational Therapy practice, theory, or education.

Ph.D Programs are offered in Full-time and Part-time.

Graduates with a Ph.D. in Occupational Therapy may pursue various career paths, including:

- Research positions in academia or research institutions.
- Faculty positions in Occupational Therapy programs.
- Leadership roles in healthcare organizations.
- Consultation and advocacy roles related to policy and practices.

Difference between B.Sc. (Occupational Therapy) and Bachelors of Occupational Therapy?

- **B.Sc. in Occupational Therapy:**
  - A "B.Sc. in Occupational Therapy" typically refers to a Bachelor of Science degree program with a major in Occupational Therapy.
  - B.Sc is a Science degree program offered in some foreign countries with a duration of 3 years.
  - Graduates of a B.Sc. in Occupational Therapy program receive a Bachelor of Science degree.
- **Bachelor of Occupational Therapy (BOT):**
  - A "Bachelor of Occupational Therapy" (BOT) program is a more specialized professional degree program that focuses exclusively on Occupational Therapy coursework.
  - The Occupational Therapy curriculum focuses on clinical practice in Occupational Therapy with a duration of 4 years and 6 months complusory rotatory internship.
  - Graduates of a BOT program is often eligible to apply for licensure as Occupational Therapists and practice in the field.

How much does Occupational Therapist earn?

The salary of Occupational Therapists in India can vary based on factors such as location, experience, education, and the specific employer. Please keep in mind that salary figures can change over time due to economic factors and evolving healthcare policies. Here is a general salary range for Occupational Therapists in India:

- **Entry-Level Salary:**
  - Occupational Therapists in India can expect an entry-level salary ranging from approximately INR 3 lakh to INR 6 lakh per annum. The actual salary may vary by location and the specific healthcare facility.

- **Experienced Occupational Therapists:**
  - Occupational Therapists with several years of experience and expertise may earn higher salaries, ranging from INR 6 lakh to INR 10 lakh or more per annum.

• How do I know if my child needs Occupational Therapy?

- If you or anyone supporting your child's health or education (e.g., teacher, speech pathologist, doctor, paediatrician) is concerned about your child's development or they are struggling with their daily activities, Occupational Therapy consultation may be able to help them.
- 'Daily activities' can range from focusing and learning at school, tying their shoelaces, making new friends, participating in sports, toileting, doing their homework, eating dinner — any part of their daily life.

• What is the scope of Occupational Therapy?

Occupational Therapy services are provided to clients across the life course. Practitioners work in collaboration with clients to address occupational needs and issues in areas such as mental health; work and industry; participation in education; rehabilitation, disability, and participation; productive aging; and health and wellness.

• Occupational Therapy the right carrier path for you?

YES, Occupational Therapy is an promising career choice for anyone who wants to help patients with their functional needs. With its holistic approach, flexibility, creativity, and high demand, Occupational Therapy offers a rewarding and fulfilling career path. If you're considering a career in healthcare, be sure to explore the many opportunities available in the field of Occupational Therapy.

- **OT a demanding Job?**

YES, Occupational Therapy is a demanding Job. Occupational Therapy help people recover from physical injuries and teach people motor and mobility skills. This can be a rewarding career for dedicated individuals who enjoy working with people, but becoming one can take hard work and time. Occupational Therapy offers a wide variety of scope of practice.

- **What is the future of Occupational Therapy in India?**

Occupational Therapy is a growing field in India, with an increasing demand for trained professionals to help individuals with disabilities, injuries, and illnesses participate in the activities of daily living. The future of Occupational Therapy in India is expected to be very promising, as the population ages and the number of people with disabilities increases. Overall, the future for Occupational Therapy in India looks bright, as there will be a growing need for Occupational Therapists to help individuals achieve their maximum level of independence and participation in daily life.

- **What is the role of an Occupational Therapist in a healthcare team, and how do they collaborate with other professionals?**

Occupational Therapists are essential members of healthcare teams, focusing on enhancing patients' functional abilities and quality of life. Their collaborative approach ensures that patients receive comprehensive care addressing physical, cognitive, emotional, and social aspects of their well-being. Effective communication and teamwork among healthcare professionals are key to providing the best possible care to patients.

- **Can Occupational Therapist do private practice?**

Yes, Occupational Therapy is an Independent Healthcare Profession, so they can do independent practice. Occupational Therapist are expertise in diagnostic procedure and intervention planning relevant to their Clinical Practice and reasoning.

- **Whether Occupational Therapy is an Allied Health or Healthcare Profession?**

Occupational Therapy is a Healthcare Profession according to the National Commission for Allied and Healthcare Professions Act, 2021.

- **What is Occupational Therapy otherwise known as?**

Occupational Therapy is otherwise called as Ergomedicine meaning Ergo = Work.

- **What does an Occupational Therapist Do?**

Occupational Therapist deal with both physically and mentally challenged people and individuals struggling with day-to-day activities to achieve maximum functional independence by using meaningful and purposeful therapeutic activities.

- **Can Occupational Therapist use the prefix "Dr" to their name?**

Yes, Occupational Therapy Graduates registered under All India Occupational Therapists' Association (AIOTA) can use the prefix "Dr" to their name. AIOTA is the only Professional body for Occupational Therapy Profession in India, and it is one of the constituent members of World Federation of Occupational Therapists (WFOT), recognized by World Health Organization (WHO).

www.ingramcontent.com/pod-product-compliance
Ingram Content Group UK Ltd.
Pitfield, Milton Keynes, MK11 3LW, UK
UKHW060359300726
14090UKWH00001B/19

* 9 7 9 8 8 9 1 8 6 4 3 5 1 *